VITAL QUESTIONS
TO ASK IN THE ER

VITAL QUESTIONS TO ASK IN THE ER

Theresa Spruill, PA-C

Level II Trauma Center
Good Samaritan Hospital
Suffern, New York

Michael S. Lippe, MD, FACEP

Director, Department of Emergency Medicine
Good Samaritan Hospital
Suffern, New York

Blackwell
Publishing

©2002 by Blackwell Science, Inc.
A Blackwell Publishing Company

Editorial Offices:
Commerce Place, 350 Main Street, Malden, Massachusetts 02148, USA
Osney Mead, Oxford OX2 0EL, England
25 John Street, London WC1N 2BS, England
23 Ainslie Place, Edinburgh EH3 6AJ, Scotland
54 University Street, Carlton, Victoria 3053, Australia

Other Editorial Offices:
Blackwell Wissenschafts-Verlag GmbH, Kurfürstendamm 57, 10707 Berlin, Germany
Blackwell Science KK, MG Kodenmacho Building, 7-10 Kodenmacho
  Nihombashi, Chuo-ku, Tokyo 104, Japan
Iowa State University Press, A Blackwell Science Company, 2121 S. State Avenue,
  Ames, Iowa 50014-8300, USA

Distributors:

The Americas
  Blackwell Publishing
  c/o AIDC
  P.O. Box 20
  50 Winter Sport Lane
  Williston, VT 05495-0020
  (Telephone orders: 800-216-2522;
      fax orders: 802-864-7626)

Outside North America and Australia
  Blackwell Science, Ltd.
  c/o Marston Book Services, Ltd.
  P.O. Box 269
  Abingdon
  Oxon OX14 4YN
  England
  (Telephone orders: 44-01235-465500;
      fax orders: 44-01235-465555)

Australia
  Blackwell Science Pty, Ltd.
  54 University Street
  Carlton, Victoria 3053
  (Telephone orders: 03-9347-0300;
      fax orders: 03-9349-3016)

Acquisitions: Beverly Copland
Development: Julia Casson
Production: Debra Lally
Manufacturing: Lisa Flanagan
Marketing Manager: Kathleen Mulcahy
Cover design by Gary Ragaglia
Interior design by Gallagher
Typeset by Gallagher
Printed and bound by Edwards Brothers/North Carolina

Printed in the United States of America
02 03 04 05 5 4 3 2 1

The Blackwell Science logo is a trade mark of Blackwell Science Ltd.,
registered at the United Kingdom Trade Marks Registry

Library of Congress Cataloging-in-Publication Data
Spruill, Theresa.
   Vital questions to ask in the ER / by Theresa Spruill, Michael S. Lippe.
      p. ; cm.
   ISBN 0-632-04668-6 (pbk.)
   1. Emergency medicine—Handbooks, manuals, etc. 2. Medical history taking—
Handbooks, manuals, etc.
   [DNLM: 1. Emergency Treatment—methods. 2. Emergencies. 3. Medical
History Taking—methods. WB 105 S927v 2002] I. Lippe, Michael S. II. Title.
   RC86.8 .S685 2002
   616.02'5—dc21

                                             2001008594

CONTENTS

	Preface	vii
	Reviewers	viii
1	Abdominal Pain	1
2	Altered Mental Status	7
3	Ankle Injuries	9
4	Back Pain	11
5	Bites	15
6	Burns	17
7	Calf Pain	19
8	Chest Pain	21
9	Constipation, Diarrhea, Hematemesis, and Melena	26
10	Cough	31
11	Depression, Anxiety, and Suicide Attempt	35
12	Difficulty Breathing	37
13	Dizziness	40
14	Ear Complaints	43
15	Edema	46
16	Epistaxis	48
17	Eye Complaints	50
18	Fever	54
19	Headache	58
20	Hematuria	63

21	Joint Pain	65
22	Lacerations and Abrasions	68
23	Motor Vehicle Accident	70
24	Nausea and Vomiting	72
25	Needlestick	75
26	Oral Complaints, Teeth, and Gingiva	76
27	Rash	79
28	Seizures, Fainting, and Loss of Consciousness	82
29	Sexual Assault	86
30	Sexually Transmitted Diseases	90
31	Shoulder Pain	93
32	Sinusitis	96
33	Sore Throat	98
34	Syncope	100
35	Urinary Tract Infection and Urinary Complaints	104
36	Vaginal Bleeding	107
37	Vaginal Discharge	111
38	Vaginal Itching	114
39	Wrist Injuries	117

PREFACE

"Oops, I forgot to ask!" is not a sentence that you want to say or one that the Attending or Chief Resident wants to hear, especially when presenting your patient's history. This book was developed based on the authors' years of experience in the ER.

Vital Questions to Ask in the ER is written as a guide for the busy medical student in the emergency room. It is organized into common complaints that patients present to the emergency department, followed by a series of questions arranged in order of importance that absolutely must be asked relating to that particular complaint. In bold following the questions are rationales for the questions. Margin notes feature points to consider or keep in mind, and "Don't forget to ask" boxes contain other points to remember.

Asking the "right" questions can save lives. Every year there are thousands of legal cases filed for alleged misdiagnosis or malpractice. Many of these cases might have been avoided if, during the initial history, the right questions had been asked.

Assessment begins from the moment the patient is called into the examination area. The way that the patient walks, talks, and acts all assist in arriving at a working diagnosis. **This book will help the student of emergency medicine in determining which pertinent questions will lead to a quick and correct diagnosis.**

During the course of evaluation, the physical condition of the emergency room patient may deteriorate suddenly; therefore, it is imperative that the practitioner of emergency medicine be able to quickly identify pathology by asking the patient the right questions. Remember, a second chance may not present itself!

Our hope is that *Vital Questions to Ask in the ER* will become a permanent part of your lab coat!

REVIEWERS

James Fletcher
Class of 2003
Eastern Virginia Medical School

Jon Gottlieb
Class of 2002
University of Miami School of Medicine

Carrie Quinn, MD
Class of 2001
Tufts University

Victor Rodriguez
Class of 2003
Tufts University

ABDOMINAL PAIN

1. How long have you had symptoms?

[Two to 12 hours after ulcer perforation the initial pain may subside and the patient may look subjectively better. Abdominal pain associated with tainted food should also be considered. Time of onset may indicate severity of disease.]

A history of indigestion, "gastritis," or flatulence may occur a few hours before onset of appendicitis or may occur over a period of a few months, as in ovarian cancer.

2. Any nausea, vomiting, diarrhea, or constipation?

[Be careful here, because all symptoms may not occur simultaneously. In fact, they may not be present at all.]

3. What did the vomit look like?

[In severe obstruction, vomitus becomes yellowish to feculent whereas hyperemesis vomitus may be regurgitated food or merely retching.]

Patient may have had slight attack of ignored pain before presentation to the Emergency Department.

4. Have you had any fever? Is it present all day or mostly at night?

[Temperature may often be normal during the acute phase of the attack. Patients with suspected ruptured ectopic pregnancy may not exhibit elevation in temperature. In intestinal obstruction, temperature may be normal or subnormal; if temperature rises and falls in a "picket fence" pattern, suspect abscess.]

5. Do you have any other medical problems?

[A number of systemic diseases may cause abdominal pain: diabetes, sickle cell disease, acute porphyria, auricular fibrillation, and congestive heart failure, to name a few.]

Always remember that your patient may present atypically and not like the textbook.

1

It is often useful to ask the patient to rate pain on scale of 1 to 10 (10 being the worst).

6. Is the pain constant or off and on?

[The character of the pain may also give clues to severity of disease, including the constant pain of perforation of gastric ulcer (which is a late sign) and abdominal pain associated with hemoperitoneum. If pain is intermittent and colicky consider renal stone, cholecystitis. Although the pain of biliary colic is steady, you should always consider the "colic's" when the patient describes the pain as intermittent, as is the case in renal colic.]

Don't forget that patients will often take over the counter preparations like Tylenol or even spare antibiotics they have had in the house. This may mask fever.

7. Does the pain go anywhere else?

[Very important question. The response is often instrumental in arriving at a correct diagnosis. For instance, radiation to testicles, as is sometimes seen with appendicitis or renal colic; pain referred to right subscapular region in cholecystitis, perforated duodenal ulcer; or left shoulder pain from hemoperitoneum secondary to ectopic pregnancy.]

8. Can you describe the pain for me?

[The response to this question may indicate severity and the nature of pathology, like the excruciating pain often associated with pancreatitis.]

Watch your patient closely. Body posture may also give clues to pathology.

9. Was the pain gradual or sudden?

[The patient's response to this question will also aid in predicting severity of pathology. But be careful! The early stages of severe pathology may present quite benign. Also, a thorough history may reveal that the patient has had several "mini" attacks of pain or long history of "indigestion."]

10. Does the pain occur particularly before or after meals?

[In duodenal ulcer, the pain occurs 2–3 hours after taking food and is relieved by taking food.]

11. Did the pain wake you out of sleep?

[Ruptured ectopic pregnancy, perforation of gastric or duodenal ulcer, and abdominal aneurysm may all awaken patient from sleep.]

12. Does the pain go into your groin?

[Commonly seen in nephrolithiasis, aortic aneurysm, appendicitis, or ovarian torsion.]

13. Have you had fainting or dizziness?

[If the patient fell down or fainted consider perforation of gastric or duodenal ulcer, acute pancreatitis, ruptured aneurysm, or ruptured ectopic pregnancy.]

14. Any history of chest pain?

[Secondary to nerve innervation, many abdominal processes are felt in the chest. *Always rule out myocardial infarct.*]

15. Do you have any pain in your shoulders?

[Ruptured ectopic pregnancy or any process that leads to extravasation of fluid into the peritoneal cavity. Perforated ulcer may elicit right shoulder pain. Pain felt in both shoulders from onset of attack is suggestive of a perforation of anterior wall of stomach.]

16. Any history of back pain?

[Consider nephrolithiasis or other kidney disorders. Patients with dissecting aneurysm will often complain of severe back pain.]

17. Have you had any shortness of breath with pain?

[Shallow respirations may occur secondarily to perforation of gastric or duodenal ulcer or rupture of esophagus, or abdominal pain may also be referred from cardiac origin.]

18. Any history of trauma? Have you been wrestling?

[Consider visceral injury secondary to blunt trauma.]

19. Were you feeling well before this?

[Pain of perforation is sudden in onset and patient may be feeling well one moment then severely ill the next.]

Always ask the patient about over the counter preparations.

Before considering pelvic inflammatory disease, be sure of patient's sexual history. If patient has not been sexually active for an extended time, the likelihood of pelvic inflammatory disease is zero.

Patients with normal pregnancy may experience dizziness.

> Always keep anatomy in mind.

20. Does any particular position make the pain better or worse?

[Pain of rupture of the esophagus is usually aggravated by lying flat and relieved by sitting.]

21. Have you had any recent surgery or procedures?

[In women who have undergone recent cervical or uterine manipulation rule out uterine perforation. Keep obstruction in mind if the history is more remote and patient has had prior abdominal procedures.]

> Patient may also be losing weight secondarily to stress.

22. Have you noticed any change in the color of your bowel movements? Have you noticed any blood?

23. Have you had any previous abdominal surgery?

[Previous abdominal surgery may lead to obstruction or ectopic pregnancy.]

24. Any change in size of the abdomen?

[Consider obstipation, megs syndrome, ovarian cancer and intestinal obstruction.]

> In assessing abdominal pain, also be on the lookout for emotional factors.

25. Have you had these or similar symptoms before?

[With a complete history you can ascertain whether patient has been having "gas," frequent indigestion, or history of vague abdominal discomfort.]

26. Have you had unusual amounts of gas or belching?

[A history of flatulence is frequently seen in appendicitis.]

> The term "bowel movement" is nice and professional, but some patients respond better to "cocky" or "poop."

27. Any weight loss? And over how long?

[Before the alarm bells go off, consider also the weight loss that may be associated with hyperemesis, neoplasm of digestive tract and ovarian cancer.]

28. Any problems making urine? Does it hurt or burn? Have you noticed any blood in the urine?

[Consider renal colic, urinary tract infection and nephrolithiasis. *Do not forget menstruation!*]

29. Are you taking any medications?

[Of particular concern are digoxin and diuretics. Consider ischemia. Also consider over the counter preparations like laxatives or herbal remedies.]

> You should consider relatively benign processes before entertaining the worst.

30. Have you recently had any fast food or food that you did not cook?

[Salmonella and shigella may produce nausea, vomiting, abdominal pain and diarrhea.]

31. When was your last normal period?

[Ectopic pregnancy and incomplete or threatened abortion all can elicit abdominal pain.]

> Ask if menses are normal. Many women will develop painful cysts on ovaries at time of menses.

32. Any vaginal bleeding or spotting that is not normal?

[Always rule out pregnancy or pain from degenerating fibroids.]

33. Any abnormal vaginal discharge?

[Here you want to keep in mind incubation period of gonorrhea and chlamydia, which are most common causes of salpingitis and secondary abdominal pain. Although abnormal discharge may be absent in both cases, a positive response to this question should lead you to do cervical cultures.]

> Salpingitis is almost always bilateral.

34. Have you had any pain during sex?

[Dyspareunia may indicate salpingitis.]

35. Any history of cysts or fibroid uterus?

[If the woman has history of leiomyoma, degenerating fibroids may present as acute abdomen.]

> Before considering STD, be sure patient has not had total abdominal hysterectomy, bilateral salpingoopherectomy. Ask about laxatives.

36. Do you normally get pain at the time of your period?

[Consider simple dysmenorrhea.]

37. When was the last time you had sex?

[Consider incubation period for gonorrhea and chlamydia and the relationship to salpingitis.]

38. Is anyone else at home sick with the cold or flu?

With the advent of the World Wrestling Federation there will be more abdominal trauma, especially in childdren and teens.

Remember that pregnant women get appendicitis, too. The appendix is often higher up in the abdomen.

Unfortunately, there are more cases of spousal abuse. Always keep your index of suspicion up.

39. Can you show me with one finger where the pain began?

[The pain may have begun in one abdominal region; however, by the time the patient is evaluated in the Emergency Department, location may have changed or radiated. For example, acute pancreatitis may begin in the central abdomen before localizing.]

40. Were you doing anything in particular when pain began?

[If pain occurred during coitus (in females) consider ruptured ovarian cyst; consider abdominal hernia if weight lifting or moving heavy objects. Though rare, rupture of the rectus muscle may follow sudden muscular effort like severe coughing.]

DON'T FORGET TO ASK:

- Duration and onset of symptoms
- Fever, nausea, vomiting, diarrhea, or constipation
- Does pain radiate?
- Medication history, including oral contraceptives, herbal preparations, and over the counter preparations
- History of shortness of breath

ALTERED MENTAL STATUS

1. **Does the patient have any significant past medical history?**

   [Consider seizure disorder, postictal states, diabetes, acute delirious states, Reye's syndrome, hypertension, or thyroid disease.]

2. **Is the patient taking any medications?**

   [The list of medications that can cause changes in mental status are numerous. However, the most common are barbiturates, benzodiazepines, anxiolytics, opiates, MAO inhibitors, cardiac glycosides, and salicylates.]

3. **Does the patient take any drugs?**

   [Narcan is recommended for patients with altered mental status of unknown cause.]

4. **Is the patient getting better or worse?**

   [This information becomes important especially in the elderly patient, in whom urosepsis may be the cause. Also consider dehydration, check chemistry, or consider a bleed.]

5. **Any known history of trauma or fall?**

   [Exercise caution in patients with suspected C-spine injury.]

6. **Did the symptoms come on gradually or suddenly?**

   [A gradual decline in mental status may indicate a metabolic cause or a space-occupying lesion. Remember also that the patient may have had a previous fall or injury that they did not report; this becomes important when a bleed is suspected.]

7. **Any history of fever?**

   [Consider an infectious process like encephalitis or meningitis.]

8. **Has the patient had a recent history of headache that is out of the ordinary?**

   [Rule out subdural hematoma, cerebrovascular accident, cerebral embolism, or space-occupying lesion.]

9. **Has the patient taken any *new* medications?**

   [Rule out medication toxicity, especially with digoxin and Librium, where the serum levels must be carefully controlled.]

DON'T FORGET TO ASK:

- Any significant past medical history?
- Did symptoms come on gradually or suddenly?
- Any history of fever?
- Medication history
- History of trauma

ANKLE INJURIES

1. What were you doing when this happened?

[Ankle injuries occur from inversion, eversion, dorsiflexion, and plantarflexion. Basketball is the most common reported sports activity that causes ankle sprains.]

2. Do you remember the position of your foot when you injured it?

[If the patient reports that the foot was in dorsiflexion, external rotation, or eversion, this should alert you to consider other injuries, such as high ankle sprain or fracture.]

3. After the initial injury, did the pain get better?

[A dorsiflexion injury that improves suddenly may indicate rupture of the superior peroneal retinaculum.]

4. Have you been able to walk on it?

[Patients who have a lateral ankle injury that did not restrict their activity immediately after the injury have mild to moderate ligamentous damage. Patients who are unable to bear weight may have sustained complete rupture of the ligamentous structures or fractures.]

5. Have you ever injured this ankle before? How many times?

[Patients with a chronically unstable ankle initially may present with an acute ankle injury. Frequency of injury can provide information about the chronicity of the ankle instability.]

6. Have you noticed any swelling or discoloration?

[Ecchymosis may or may not be present; with more severe injuries, it is almost always noted. Deformity of the ankle often indicates fracture or dislocation.]

7. Are you allergic to any medication?

[Antibiotic therapy may be necessary, especially in the event of open fracture.]

8. When was your last tetanus shot?

[Again, this is very important if there is suspected open fracture.]

9. Do you have any medical problems?

[Patients with a history of diabetes, who are immunosuppressed, or with a history of collagen vascular disease are susceptible to delayed wound healing.]

10. Are you taking any medication?

[Of particular importance is corticosteroids.]

DON'T FORGET TO ASK:

- Mechanism of injury
- Position of the foot at the time of injury
- Past medical history
- If patient is able to bear weight

BACK PAIN

1. **Any history of trauma? Were you hit at all? Did you fall?**

   [The most common cause of back pain is trauma, either from muscle strain, a fall, or a "pull."]

   Onset of pain after exertion is usually due to muscular or ligamentous strain but may also be associated with stress fractures or compression fractures.

2. **What were you doing when pain started?**

   [This is closely related to the first question. If the onset of symptoms can be closely correlated with some physical activity and serious pathology like acute myocardial infarction or rupture of an aneurysm has been ruled out, the symptoms are more than likely related to a musculoskeletal process.]

3. **Is the pain only in one spot or does it go somewhere else?**

   [Back pain radiating to the groin may indicate nephrolithiasis; always keep in mind the possibility of dissecting aneurysm. In some instances, the pain associated with cholecystitis will start in the back before localizing to the right upper quadrant. Lower back pain that radiates to the buttock and down the leg may indicate sciatica.]

4. **Have you had this before?**

   [This becomes important in patients with "chronic back pain" when considering treatment modalities and pain management.]

5. **Are you taking any medications?**

   [Ask about anticoagulants and nonsteroidal anti-inflammatory drugs. Patients may also have self-medicated at home, thus masking the actual severity of the pain and condition.]

6. **Do you have any medical problems that a doctor is treating you for?**

[Consider hypertension, diabetes, arthritis, or collagen vascular disease. A past history of cancer, either prostate or urinary, raises the suspicion of a metastatic lesion to the spine.]

7. **Have you had any abdominal pain?**

[Again, take the entire medical history into consideration. Cholecystitis or abdominal aortic aneurysm may initially present with back pain.]

8. **Have you had any pain, burning, or difficulty urinating?**

[Patients with upper urinary tract infection or those brewing a pyelonephritis may complain of back pain.]

9. **Any nausea or vomiting?**

[This may indicate a gastrointestinal origin of the pain, particularly if it is the initial presenting symptom. Patients who have pyelonephritis are generally toxic looking and have vomiting.]

10. **Have you been working out or wrestling?**

[Again, rule out a musculoskeletal process.]

11. **Have you noticed any blood in the urine? What color is the urine?**

[Patients with renal involvement may complain of hematuria, or "dark urine," associated with the back pain. Consider urinary tract infection, nephrolithiasis, or trauma. Don't forget to ask the patient if she is menstruating or nearing the end of her menses.]

12. **Does it hurt to take a deep breath?**

[A pleuritic component may suggest pneumothorax, pneumonia, muscle strain, or rib fracture. Let the rest of your history be your guide.]

13. **Any history of chest pain since the development of back pain?**

    [Many thoracic and gastrointestinal processes may present with back pain: consider myocardial infarction or gastroesophageal reflux disease.]

14. **Have you had any weakness or loss of strength in limbs?**

    [Neurologic findings may indicate a radiculopathy. Elderly patients with a history of minimal trauma may have lumbar or thoracic stress fracture.]

15. **Have you had any fever?**

    [Always consider an infectious process.]

16. **Did the pain come on suddenly or gradually?**

    [Sudden excruciating back pain without a history of trauma may indicate aneurysm. Pain of insidious onset may arise from spinal stenosis, spondylolisthesis, neoplasms of prostate or urinary tract, or infection.]

17. **Have you had any problems with bowel or bladder function that is not *normal* since the onset of back pain?**

    [In patients who present with back pain and recent onset of constipation or incontinence, consider cauda equina syndrome.]

18. **Any history of fibroids or painful periods?**

    [Patients with a history of leiomyoma may complain of lower back pain.]

19. **Is the pain made worse by movement?**

    [Patients with spinal stenosis may complain of back and leg pain that is increased by walking or standing.]

20. **Does rest make it better?**

    [If the pain is alleviated by rest, consider spinal tumor, fracture, infection, or referred pain from visceral structures.]

DON'T FORGET TO ASK:

- History of trauma
- Fever
- Did the pain begin somewhere else and localize to the back?
- Abdominal pain
- Significant past medical history

BITES

1. **When did this happen?**

   [When patients seek care more than 12 hours after the injury, there is a greater chance of infection.]

2. **Do you know if the immunization of the animal is up to date?**

   [Properly immunized domestic animals do not transmit rabies.]

3. **When was your last tetanus shot?**

   [If tetanus immunization was more than 5 years ago, a standard booster dose of tetanus-diphtheria should be given.]

4. **How did this happen?**

   [Most clenched-fist injuries result in trauma-tized tissue seeded by oral bacteria and often involve tendons, joints, and bones.]

5. **What kind of dog was it?**

   [The jaws of large dogs like rottweilers can exert more than 250 psi of pressure, causing substantial crush trauma.]

6. **Any history of allergy? What is the reaction?**

   [This is very important when considering pro-phylactic antibiotic coverage.]

7. **Do you have any history of liver disease?**

   [Bite infections are more severe in patients with liver disease, active or chronic hepatitis, and alcohol consumption.]

8. **Have you had any surgery on your belly?**

   [Like previous splenectomy.]

9. **Did you have any swelling in the area before the bite?**

   [These patients are at greater risk of serious infection.]

10. **On a scale of 1 to 10, with 10 being the worst, how bad is the pain?**

    [In patients who complain of pain out of proportion to the severity of the injury, especially when it involves the hand or near a joint, suspect joint penetration or early septic arthritis or osteomyelitis.]

11. **Can you move the hand?**

    [A significant decrease in range of motion may indicate nerve or tendon disruption.]

12. **Are you taking any medications?**

    [Particularly anticoagulants, nonsteroidals, aspirin, or vitamin E.]

13. **Have you had any fever or chills?**

    [Some patients may delay treatment and subsequently develop a systemic infection.]

14. **Were you petting the animal and being friendly to it?**

    [An unprovoked attack by an animal with bizarre behavior should arouse suspicion that it might be rabid.]

15. **Do you have any medical problems?**

    [Diabetes mellitus, chronic edema, lupus, or presence of a prosthetic limb or joint.]

DON'T FORGET TO ASK:

- Mechanism of injury
- When did the injury occur?
- Any history of fever
- History of decreased range of motion
- Immunization of the animal
- Tetanus immunization

BURNS

1. How did this happen?

[Treatment modalities differ depending on the mechanism of injury, including flash burns, electric, or scalding. Flame-induced injuries produce full thickness injuries and may be associated with inhalation injuries. Seventy-five percent of patients involved in fires in an enclosed space have inhalation injuries.]

All burns should be checked in 24 hours.

2. Do you have any significant past medical history?

[Diabetes, steroid use, immunosuppression— all are implicated in delayed wound healing and the necessity of antibiotic therapy.]

3. When was your last tetanus?

[If tetanus immunization was more than 5 years before the injury, a standard booster dose of tetanus-diphtheria should be given.]

4. Any history of headache, nausea, or vomiting?

[Consider carbon monoxide poisoning.]

5. Do you have any allergies?

[Remember you may have to administer antibiotic therapy.]

6. Have you had any shortness of breath or difficulty breathing?

[This may indicate respiratory involvement.]

7. Was there any chemical exposure?

[The management of chemical burns depends on the agent involved. Every effort should be made to find the agent. Patients will often bring the product with them. Look on the container and call the company.]

17

DON'T FORGET TO ASK:

- Mechanism of injury
- Tetanus history
- History of allergies
- Significant past medical history

CALF PAIN

1. How long have you had this pain?

[In acute arterial occlusion, the pain is abrupt, whereas patients with varicose veins may complain of pain present over an extended period of time. In arteriosclerosis obliterans, the pain is also gradual and progressive in onset.]

In arteriosclerosis obliterans, the pain rarely occurs with standing or sitting.

2. Is the pain felt in both legs or just one?

[Unilateral calf pain is of more concern. Consider the rest of the history. Unilateral leg pain is a strong indicator of deep vein thrombosis.]

3. Do you have any medical problems for which a doctor is treating you?

[Patients who are obese or have a sedentary life-style may be susceptible to the development of deep vein thrombosis. Also, patients with a history of hypertension, diabetes, myocardial infarction, antithrombin 111, protein S and C deficiency. Ask about any history of malignancy, particularly breast or lung.]

4. Have you had fever or chills?

[Fever is present in superficial thrombophlebitis. Also consider cellulitis.]

5. Does walking make the pain worse?

[In deep vein thrombosis, the pain is made worse by standing or walking.]

6. Does any particular position make the pain better?

[In deep vein thrombosis and varicose veins, elevation of the affected extremity will relieve symptoms.]

19

7. **Are you taking any medications?**

   [Patients taking oral contraceptives or who are on estrogen replacement therapy may be at increased risk for developing deep vein thrombosis. Also ask about cardiac medications, including anticoagulants.]

8. **Does it hurt to touch?**

   [Pain associated with light touch may indicate superficial thrombosis or cellulitis. Pain that is felt on deep palpation is more likely deep vein thrombosis.]

9. **Have you noticed any swelling?**

   [In post-thrombotic syndrome, swelling is worse at the end of the day, whereas in lymphedema, swelling will subside at night.]

10. **Does the pain go anywhere else?**

    [In lymphedema, swelling starts in the foot and progresses proximally.]

11. **Has there been any discoloration or redness?**

    [This is indicative of trauma, cellulitis, superficial thrombophlebitis, or lymphedema.]

12. **Do you sense a "heaviness" in the leg(s)?**

    [This is a typical symptom with varicose veins.]

13. **Any shortness of breath or dyspnea?**

    [Patients with leg pain should also be assessed for signs and symptoms of pulmonary embolism.]

14. **Have you taken any *new* drugs or medications?**

    [As in allergic lymphedema.]

DON'T FORGET TO ASK:

- Significant past medical history
- Do you smoke?
- Any history of fever?
- Does anything make the pain better?

CHEST PAIN

1. **How long have you had the pain?**

   [Patients with angina may report pain or discomfort that generally lasts for several minutes, whereas patients with true myocardial infarction usually have more than 20 minutes of discomfort.]

2. **Can you describe to me what the pain feels like?**

   [The classic symptom of acute myocardial infarction is described as "crushing" or "pressure."]

3. **Does it hurt you to take a deep breath?**

   [Patients who complain of pleuritic chest pain may have pneumonia or pericarditis.]

4. **Have you recently had a cold, flu, or fever?**

   [Localized pleuritic chest pain that is associated with cough or fever may be representative of pneumonia.]

5. **What were you doing when you first noticed the pain?**

   [Strenuous activity may lead to cardiac oxygen depletion and subsequent ischemia.]

6. **Does the pain stay in your chest or go to any other part of your body?**

   [In acute myocardial infarct, the pain may radiate to the arm, jaw, or neck. The pain of pericarditis may also be referred to the neck.]

7. **Have you had any nausea or vomiting?**

   [Nausea or vomiting may be present in acute posterior wall myocardial infarction.]

> Treat the patient, not the laboratory values.

> Watch your patient for clues to his or her illness; invariably, body language will assist you with diagnosis.

> Keep in mind the patient's emotional state. Anxiety can also cause chest pain.

8. **Have you noticed any increase in gas or burping?**

   [A history of flatulence is common when the cause of the chest pain has a gastrointestinal origin. Remember that these symptoms may also occur in ischemia.]

9. **Have you had this pain before?**

   [A history of frequent chest pain that resolves with intervention may indicate a gastrointestinal component or anxiety.]

10. **Do you have any medical problems for which you are under a doctor's care?**

    [Also consider spinal arthritis. Always consider "other" medical problems in which the symptoms may radiate to the chest.]

11. **Is the pain worse at night?**

    [Patients with a history of gastric ulcer disease may say that the pain is worse at night.]

12. **Any abdominal or back pain with the chest pain?**

    [The pain associated with aortic dissection often radiates to the back. Also consider intra-abdominal origin of the pain like cholecystitis, or peptic or gastric ulcer disease.]

13. **Does lying down or any particular position make pain better or worse?**

    [In pericarditis pain becomes sharper and more left sided in the supine position and decreased when patient sits up right or leaning forward.]

14. **Have you been wrestling, boxing, or doing heavy work lately?**

    [Consider cardiac contusion, chest wall contusion, or muscle strain.]

15. **Are you a smoker?**

    [Patients who smoke are at an increased risk for coronary artery disease. In mediastinal emphysema, patients may complain of pain that radiates from the substernal area to the shoulders.]

16. **Can you make the pain return if you touch the area?**

[In costochondritis, the patient will have reproducible pain.]

17. **When you first noticed it, where did the pain begin?**

[In angina pectoris, the pain is often described as a "discomfort" and is substernal rather than the frank precordial pain associated with myocardial infarction. The pain that is associated with acute dissection of the aorta is *extremely* severe and localized to the center of the chest or back.]

18. **Did the pain come on suddenly or gradually?**

[Pain due to acute dissection of the aorta is usually extremely severe and localized to the center of the chest and lasts for hours and may not respond to analgesics.]

19. **Did you take anything to alleviate the pain? Did it help?**

[The pain of gastric or duodenal ulcer is epigastric and may be relieved by antacids. The pain associated with aortic dissection may not respond to analgesics. In contrast to angina, the pain of acute myocardial infarction is not relieved by rest or coronary dilator drugs and may require increased narcotics.]

20. **Are you currently taking any medications?**

[Medications containing pseudoephedrine may cause a sensation of heaviness. Also, ask about herbal preparations containing Gurana or Mah Haung because they may cause palpitations or chest discomfort.]

21. **Have you had the feeling that your heart is beating too fast or skipping beats?**

[Consider anxiety disorder. Ask about caffeine intake or diet pills.]

22. Is there any heart disease, diabetes, or stroke in the family? Any family history at all?

[Patients with a significant family history of coronary artery disease or diabetes are at an increased risk of myocardial infarction.]

23. Does it hurt or is the skin over the area sensitive? Did you notice any tingling over the chest before the pain?

[Consider herpes zoster or shingles.]

24. Any breast pain?

[The pain of acute myocardial infarct may be experienced as breast pain.]

25. Are you taking any over the counter drugs, including cough syrup?

[Many over the counter preparations can cause palpitations.]

26. Does the pain occur at rest also?

[In esophageal spasm or unstable angina chest pain, chest pain may occur at rest or occur following less and less activity.]

27. Did the pain wake you from sleep?

[Variant (Prinzmetal's) angina may awaken patient from sleep.]

28. Have you had any shortness of breath? Do you have shortness of breath upon minor exertion?

[Shortness of breath upon minor exertion with associated chest pain may indicate myocardial infarction, congestive heart failure, or pneumothorax.]

29. Have you had any fainting or dizziness?

[In hypertrophic cardiomyopathy, chest pain may be associated with dyspnea, syncope, or sudden death.]

30. Do you have a history of very heavy periods or fibroids?

[Menorrhagia may lead to anemia and a feeling of chest discomfort.]

31. **Any history of trauma? Have you taken a fall or were you hit?**

    [Consider cardiac contusion as a cause of chest pain.]

32. **Can you show me exactly where the pain started?**

    [Angina pain is characteristically substernal rather than precordial.]

33. **Did you notice the pain after eating a particular food or drinking something?**

    [Consider gastric ulcer disease.]

34. **Is the pain particularly worse after meals?**

    [In duodenal ulcer, the pain may occur 2–3 hours after eating.]

35. **Does it hurt to swallow?**

    [Esophageal perforation can cause severe retrosternal chest pain that is made worse by swallowing. In pericarditis, substernal chest pain may be increased by swallowing and breathing.]

36. **Does the pain stay in your chest or does it go to another part of the body?**

    [In acute myocardial infarction the pain may radiate to the arm, jaw, or neck. The pain of pericarditis may also be referred to the neck.]

DON'T FORGET TO ASK:

- Where pain started and if it radiates
- Significant past medical history
- History of shortness of breath or dyspnea
- Associated symptoms of nausea, vomiting, or diaphoresis
- Associated abdominal or back pain
- History of syncope

CONSTIPATION, DIARRHEA, HEMATEMESIS, AND MELENA

1. **When was the last time that you had a bowel movement? Is that normal for you?**

   [Normalcy in bowel habits varies from person to person. Be sure to ask the patient about his or her *normal* pattern.]

2. **How often are you going?**

   [Frequent watery stools may lead to volume depletion and associated symptoms of weakness, fatigue, or syncope. Diarrhea persisting for weeks may be a manifestation of serious illness. Acute diarrhea, presumed to be viral, typically persists for 1 to 3 days.]

3. **What color is the stool? Is it black or "sticky"?**

   [Melena has an upper tract source in about 95% of cases, but it may also result from bleeding in the small bowel or right colon. Diarrhea may be clear as in cholera or grossly bloody as seen in ulcerative colitis, shigellosis, or amebiasis.]

4. **Did you notice if the stool floated?**

   [In irritable bowel syndrome, stools are apt to become thin, fragmented, or pellet-like with excessive gas and mucus.]

5. **Did you notice any *obvious* bleeding?**

   [Consider hemorrhoids. Hematochezia represents bleeding from the colon in about 85% of cases. Melena is usually associated with bleeding from the esophagus, stomach, or duodenum.]

6. **Is the odor particularly foul smelling?**

   [Foul-smelling stools are often produced in cases of sprue or pancreatic insufficiency.]

7. **Are you having a lot of gas with the bowel movement?**

[Small frequent bowel movements with increased flatulence is typical in irritable bowel syndrome.]

8. **Are you having difficulty holding your bowel movement?**

[This could indicate anal sphincter abnormality.]

9. **Are your bowel movements painful?**

[Anal gonorrhea can lead to rectal pain and painful bowel movements. Diverticulitis is accompanied by fever, tenesmus, and rectal urgency with pain.]

10. **Did symptoms come on gradually or suddenly?**

[Acute diarrhea in a healthy person is usually due to an infectious process. Variceal bleeding is usually abrupt and massive. Acute onset of bloody diarrhea may indicate inflammatory bowel disease or an infectious colitis. Sudden onset of constipation and tenesmus may signal the possibility of carcinoma of the rectum or sigmoid colon.]

11. **Have you had fever?**

[Ulcerative colitis, Crohn's disease, and diverticulitis may all present with temperature elevation.]

12. **Any history of loss of appetite, vomiting, or nausea?**

[Blood must remain in the gut for 8 hours to produce melena. Recent retching, or vomiting, followed by hematemesis suggests the possibility of Mallory-Weiss syndrome. Also consider mucosal disorders and endocrine disorders.]

13. Are you taking any new medications or antibiotics?

[Iron and bismuth subsalicylate can produce stools that appear black and are guaiac positive without actual gastrointestinal bleeding but are usually *not* tarry. Opiates, calcium, and antacids may cause constipation. Also, ask about ingestion of magnesium-containing antacids. And consider anticholinergic agents.]

14. How long have you had the symptoms?

[When constipation and tenesmus of recent onset are reported, the possibility of cancer of rectum or sigmoid colon must be suspected.]

15. What did you have to eat before onset of symptoms?

[Diarrhea developing within 12 hours of a meal may be due to staph exotoxin. Neurologic symptoms such as paresthesias, headache, or visual disturbances may suggest botulism or shellfish poisoning.]

16. Is anyone else at home ill?

[Bacterial diarrhea should be suspected if there is a history of simultaneous illness in family members who have shared contaminated food.]

17. Have you had any abdominal pain or cramping?

[Ulcerative colitis and Crohn's disease may begin as acute diarrhea with bloody stools and abdominal pain. Also consider gastric and duodenal ulcer, gastritis, esophagitis, and inflammatory bowel disease.]

18. Do you have anal intercourse?

[*Entamoeba histolytica* is prevalent in the male homosexual population, which produces an inflammatory colitis resembling ulcerative colitis. Also consider proctitis.]

19. Have you traveled out of the country recently?

[Giardiasis may cause prolonged watery diarrhea.]

20. **Any history of weight loss?**

   [Mucosal disorders like sprue are associated with weight loss and malodorous stools. Abdominal distention, anemia, and weight loss, with changing bowel habits, constipation, or thin stools, associated with gastrointestinal bleeding suggest malignancy in the left colon.]

21. **Any significant past medical history for which you are under a doctor's care?**

   [Chronic diarrhea may be secondary to thyrotoxicosis, diabetes mellitus, or adrenal insufficiency. Also consider blood dyscrasias, leukemia, or disseminated intravascular coagulation.]

22. **Have you taken aspirin, ibuprofen, or "blood thinners"?**

   [Patients who use nonsteroidal anti-inflammatory drugs are about three times more likely to have major gastrointestinal bleeding than nonusers.]

23. **Is there any history of alcoholism?**

   [Alcohol ingestion is frequently associated with acute gastrointestinal hemorrhage or hemorrhagic gastritis.]

24. **Have you had any straining or violent coughing?**

   [A history of violent straining coughing or blunt abdominal trauma associated with gastrointestinal bleeding may be a result of Mallory-Weiss syndrome.]

25. **Have you had any rectal pain?**

   [Rectal pain often accompanies hemorrhoids and anal fissures; proctitis seen in male homosexuals may be due to gonorrheal or mycoplasma infection.]

26. **Is the bleeding painless?**

   [Painless bleeding may arise from colonic diverticula, arterial venous malformation, and esophageal varices.]

27. Have you ever had this kind of bleeding before?

[Any previous history of gastrointestinal bleeding is important, because 60% of subsequent bleeding occurs at the same site.]

28. Have you ever had any surgery on your abdomen or stomach? Have you ever had an aneurysm?

[A history of abdominal aortic aneurysm or graft in association with gastrointestinal bleeding may indicate aortoenteric fistula.]

29. Have you had any fainting or dizziness?

[Patients with diarrhea need to be assessed for dehydration. If bleeding is suspected this may indicate anemia secondary to occult bleeding.]

30. Have you noticed any rash with the onset of diarrhea?

[May suggest typhoid.]

31. Have you any history of arthritis?

[May suggest a systemic cause of symptoms, especially inflammatory bowel disease.]

32. Any history of syncope?

[This is an indication of volume depletion secondary to dehydration or blood loss.]

DON'T FORGET TO ASK:

- Duration of symptoms
- Frequency of symptoms
- Any history of fever?
- Significant past medical history
- If the patient is taking medications
- If the patient is taking iron
- What patient had to eat before onset of symptoms
- Dizziness or syncope

COUGH

1. **How long have you had a cough?**

   [Estimating the duration of cough is key to narrowing the list of possible diagnosis. Post-nasal drip is the most common cause of chronic cough.]

Ask also about marijuana use.

2. **Does anything come up when you cough? What color?**

   [In pneumonia, sputum may be mucoid or bloody. In lung abscess, the sputum may be foul smelling.]

3. **Have you had any fever or runny nose?**

   [Pneumonia frequently follows an upper respiratory tract infection. Also consider postnasal drip.]

4. **Have you had any shortness of breath?**

   [Patients with a long history of shortness of breath and cough that is worse at night may be displaying signs of congestive heart failure. Patients with pneumonia and upper respiratory infection may also complain of cough and shortness of breath.]

5. **Does it hurt to breathe or take a deep breath?**

   [Pleuritic chest discomfort associated with cough may indicate pneumonia, spontaneous pneumothorax, or costochondritis.]

6. **Any significant medical problems?**

   [Gastroesophageal reflux, a medical history of sinusitis, hypertension, human immunodeficiency virus, sarcoidosis, and hyperthyroidism.]

31

7. **Do you smoke anything?**

   [Consider tobacco-induced cough. Also ask about marijuana use. In patients with a long history of smoking, who present with chronic cough, consider the possibility of malignancy.]

8. **Any wheezing?**

   [Patients with bronchitis, asthma, or foreign body may have cough with wheezing. Nocturnal wheezing is commonly observed in congestive heart failure.]

9. **Have you spit or coughed any blood?**

   [Patients reporting a history of hemoptysis may have pneumonia, tuberculosis, or a Mallory-Weiss tear.]

10. **Any significant weight loss?**

    [A history of chronic cough with associated weight loss may indicate malignancy or HIV infection.]

11. **Any night sweats?**

    [Consider pneumonia, tuberculosis, human immunodeficiency virus, although even the simple exertion associated with vigorous cough may elicit perspiration.]

12. **What kind of work do you do?**

    [Chemical inhalants or allergens in the work place may precipitate cough.]

13. **Have you had this cough before? When?**

    [Often cough is the sole presenting symptom in asthma. Also in gastroesophageal reflux disease without symptoms of heartburn or dyspepsia.]

14. **Are you taking any medications?**

    [Commonly, angiotensin-converting enzyme inhibitors can cause chronic cough.]

15. **Any history of frequent indigestion or heartburn?**

    [Gastroesophageal reflux disease is the third most common cause of chronic cough.]

16. **Any history of blood transfusions?**

    [May become relevant if suspecting human immunodeficiency virus.]

17. **Have you seen the child put anything into his or her mouth?**

    [In children, coughing can be caused by a foreign body located in the esophagus, stomach, external ear canal, or airway. The most common age for foreign body aspiration is 1–5 years.]

18. **Anyone else at home sick?**

    [Consider upper respiratory infection.]

19. **Any shortness of breath with the cough?**

    [Consider pneumonia, congestive heart failure, or chronic obstructive pulmonary disease.]

20. **Is the cough made worse by lying down?**

    [Patients with gastroesophageal reflux may complain that the cough is worse when lying down.]

21. **Is the cough made worse by exercise?**

    [Patients with emphysema and congestive heart failure have a long history of cough and exertional dyspnea.]

22. **Does anything make the cough worse? Is it related to exercise or position?**

    [Patients with gastroesophageal reflux or CHF may complain that the cough is worse when supine. Patients with emphysema and congestive heart failure have a long history of cough and exertional dyspnea.]

23. **Do you frequently have to "clear" your throat or swallow mucus?**

    [This finding is classic in postnasal drip.]

24. **Is the cough worse at night?**

    [Patients with asthma or congestive heart failure may complain of worsening cough at night.]

25. Any history of eczema?

[In patients with a history of cough and a history of eczema, think of asthma.]

26. Is the cough improved by taking antacids?

[If the patient has gastroesophageal reflux disease, H_2 blockers may relieve cough.]

DON'T FORGET TO ASK:

- Onset of cough
- Associated fever or chest pain
- Significant past medical history
- Is the cough productive or nonproductive?
- Any history of smoking?

DEPRESSION, ANXIETY, AND SUICIDE ATTEMPT

11

1. **What brings you to the emergency room?**

   [Let the patient give *you* the history if you suspect suicidal ideation; do not ask leading or open-ended questions.]

   > Be sure to ask about drug history.

2. **Have you ever felt this way before?**

   [Helps to establish history of depression, suicide, or anxiety.]

3. **Are you currently taking any medications?**

   [It is important to ask about psychiatric medications and compliance, because in many instances noncompliance may precipitate or exacerbate psychiatric symptoms.]

   > In the elderly or in cases of sudden change in affect, you must rule out physical, chemical, or neurologic abnormality.

4. **Are you now seeing a psychiatrist or in treatment for depression or anxiety?**

   [If the patient has a psychiatrist you may want to call her or him to get a more extensive history.]

5. **Are you now hearing or have you ever heard voices in your head?**

   [May be indication of severe depression with psychotic features or schizophrenia.]

6. **Do you feel like hurting yourself or others?**

   [The answer to this question may determine if admission is necessary.]

   > Severe anorexia and sleep disturbances that are chronic may indicate depression.

7. **How is your appetite? Are you sleeping and bathing?**

   [A decline in appetite and hygiene may be indicative of depression.]

35

8. Did something in particular happen to make you so upset?

[Emotional trauma may precipitate depression.]

9. Have you had chest pain or a feeling that your heart is beating fast?

[Consider anxiety disorder.]

10. Do you sometimes feel afraid for no reason, like something bad is gong to happen?

[Anxiety or panic disorder.]

11. How are things at home, school, work?

[Try to gain an appreciation for precipitating factors.]

12. Have you ever been hospitalized for any mental illness before?

[Previous hospitalization may indicate severity of patient's disease.]

13. Is this the first time you attempted suicide?

[The frequency of attempts is a strong indicator that patient may attempt again.]

14. How did you try to kill yourself?

[The more violent the attempt, the more likely they are to try it again.]

15. Do you know anyone who tried to commit suicide? A family member?

[It is not unusual for a surviving family member of a suicide to attempt same.]

16. Are there things you used to do that you are no longer interested in?

[Strong indicator of depression.]

DON'T FORGET TO ASK:

- Are you feeling like you want to hurt yourself or someone else?
- Are you taking any street drugs or prescription drugs?
- Are you currently seeing a psychiatrist?
- Ask about prior suicide attempts

CHAPTER 12

DIFFICULTY BREATHING

1. Any medical problems?

[Consider congestive heart failure, hypertension, diabetes, coronary artery disease, pericarditis, chronic obstructive pulmonary disease, asthma, arrhythmias, and collagen vascular disease.]

2. Do you smoke? Have you ever?

[A history of smoking increases the risk of developing heart disease. Also think of chronic bronchitis.]

3. Are you taking any new medications?

[Beta-blockers may cause dyspnea. Oral contraceptive use may predispose to thromboembolic disease, especially if the patient is also a smoker.]

4. Have you had any chest pain or discomfort?

[As with left ventricular failure, pulmonary embolus, pneumothorax, myocardial infarct or cardiomyopathies.]

5. Have you had fever?

[Patients presenting with fever, shortness of breath, or dyspnea may have pneumonia. If the patient appears especially toxic, consider sepsis.]

6. Do you have to sleep on extra pillows to alleviate the shortness of breath?

[Orthopnea is characteristic in left ventricular failure, severe cardiopulmonary disease and congestive heart failure.]

7. **Did the difficulty breathing come on suddenly or while at rest?**

   [Consider the rest of the patient's history; sudden shortness of breath may be indicative of emboli, spontaneous pneumothorax, severe cardiopulmonary disease or a noncardiopulmonary process like acidosis.]

8. **Is the shortness of breath worse at night?**

   [Nocturnal dyspnea is characteristic of ventricular failure and also gastroesophageal reflux.]

9. **Does lying down make it worse?**

   [Patients with congestive heart failure or asthma may complain that breathing is worse when lying down.]

10. **Have you seen the child put anything into his or her mouth?**

    [Cough associated with dyspnea or shortness of breath in children may indicate foreign body ingestion.]

11. **Any allergies?**

    [Seasonal allergies may cause dyspnea or exacerbate asthma.]

12. **Was there any evidence of food around the mouth?**

    [In the debilitated patient think of aspiration.]

13. **Have you noticed any swelling in feet or ankles?**

    [Consider congestive heart failure.]

14. **Any history of trauma? Did you fall or were you wrestling or hit by something in the chest?**

    [Think of pneumothorax.]

15. **Did the shortness of breath wake you from sleep?**

    [Nocturnal dyspnea is characteristic of ventricular failure and gastroesophageal reflux.]

16. **Have you had any chest pain or discomfort?**

    [Pleuritic chest pain and dyspnea may indicate pneumonia, pleurisy, myopathy, or pulmonary embolism. Also consider costochondritis.]

17. **Any frequent burping or flatulence?**

    [Increased flatulence secondary to gastro-esophageal reflux disease may cause a sensation of shortness of breath.]

18. **Any recent history of surgery?**

    [In patients who have undergone recent surgery (24–48 hours), consider pulmonary embolus or thromboembolus.]

19. **Have you noticed the shortness of breath after only minor exercise or exertion?**

    [Consider cardiac or pulmonary disease, especially congestive heart failure. Also consider anemia.]

20. **What kind of work do you do?**

    [Occupational exposure to dust, asbestos, or volatile chemicals may lead to interstitial lung disease.]

21. **Does it hurt to take a deep breath?**

    [Pleuritic chest pain and dyspnea may indicate pneumonia, pleurisy, myopathy, or pulmonary embolism. Also consider costochondritis.]

22. **How are things at home? Are there any new stresses in your life?**

    [If all medical pathology has been ruled out, consider anxiety.]

DON'T FORGET TO ASK:

- Significant past medical history
- Onset of symptoms
- History of smoking
- Medications

DIZZINESS

Vertigo is the initial complaint in approximately 5% of patients with multiple sclerosis.

The most common causes of peripheral vertigo are benign positional vertigo, acute labyrinthitis, and Ménière's disease. A rare cause may be herpes zoster oticus.

1. **Do you have any medical problems?**

   [Consider cardiac arrhythmias, cardiomyopathy, hypertension, diabetes mellitus, congestive heart failure.]

2. **Have you had a headache associated with the dizziness?**

   [Vertigo lasting for hours without significant auditory or neurologic symptoms is most commonly migrainous in origin.]

3. **Have you had this before? How often?**

   [Patients who report frequent "dizzy spells" or a feeling of being "far away" or detached from their environment or general sensations of imbalance in the absence of neurologic findings may suffer from panic or chronic anxiety disorder.]

4. **How long does this usually last?**

   [Episodes lasting for hours, with fluctuating and progressive sensorineural hearing loss and tinnitus, suggests Ménière's disease. Vertigo lasting for hours in the absence of auditory symptoms is most commonly migrainous.]

5. **Have you had nausea or vomiting?**

   [With Ménière's disease, patients may have severe nausea and vomiting during the attack.]

6. **Any recent history of cold, flu, or ear infection?**

   [Labyrinthitis may follow bacterial or viral infection.]

7. **Have you had any ringing in your ear?**

   [Ménière's disease, labyrinthitis, and multiple sclerosis are all possibilities.]

8. **Do you feel unsteady on your feet or like you're going to fall?**

   [In the presence of other neurologic symptoms with ipsilateral ataxia, this suggests brainstem stroke. Also consider degenerative or metabolic disorders.]

9. **Is the sensation worse or more noticeable when you go from lying to standing?**

   [Postural hypotension suggests hypovolemia or autonomic failure.]

10. **Are you taking any medications?**

    [The list of medications that may cause vertigo is endless; however, the worst offenders are cardiac medications. Check that digoxin level!]

11. **Did the attack come on suddenly or gradually?**

    [Cardiac syncope is often sudden, as in classic strokes, Adams attack of third-degree heart block, and pulmonary emboli.]

12. **Have you noticed any changes or disturbances in your vision?**

    [Symptoms of diplopia may suggest brainstem ischemia or infarction.]

13. **Are the symptoms made worse or better by any particular position?**

    [The onset or exacerbation of symptoms with particular head positions suggests benign positional vertigo.]

14. **Have you noticed any changes in your hearing?**

    [Consider Ménière's disease, labyrinthitis, acoustic neuroma.]

> Vertigo can occur with severe brainstem compression. The most common tumors are acoustic neuroma, meningioma, arterial venous malformations, and epidermoid cysts.

15. Any recent history of injury or trauma?

[Vertigo, associated with a history of facial or ear trauma, may suggest perilymph fistula. Always search for neurologic symptoms to rule out a bleed.]

16. Have you recently traveled by air or gone diving?

[Vertigo after injury to the ear or barotrauma.]

17. Do you feel like the room is spinning?

[In vertigo, patients have the sensation that they or their surroundings are spinning.]

18. Have you had any hearing loss on one side?

[Acoustic neuroma may present with asymmetric sensorineural hearing loss and vertigo.]

19. Does closing your eyes make dizziness worse?

[Think of Ménière's disease.]

20. Are the attacks severe?

[Vertigo related to peripheral vestibular disease is usually severe, whereas vertigo associated with central disease is quite mild.]

21. Do you smoke?

[In patients who smoke, the incidence of coronary artery disease or stroke is increased.]

DON'T FORGET TO ASK:

- About neurologic symptoms
- Significant past medical history
- History of medications, including herbal preparations
- Does positioning affect incidence?
- Any history of chest pain, dyspnea, or shortness of breath?

EAR COMPLAINTS

1. **How long have you had the pain?**

   [Patients with otitis media complain of hours to days of ear pain; also consider otitis externa, foreign body, or barotrauma.]

   > Unilateral hearing loss of sudden onset may indicate viral infection.

2. **Can you hear out of the ear? Is it muffled?**

   [Consider your entire history; this may indicate barotrauma, tympanic membrane perforation, foreign body, or cerumen impaction.]

3. **Any history of trauma? Were you playing around or hit on the face, head, or near the ear?**

   [Injuries to the head or face may result in tympanic membrane perforation.]

   > Gradual hearing loss may indicate otosclerosis schwannoma of acoustic nerve or Ménière's disease.

4. **Have you used cotton swabs or put anything into the ear?**

   [Consider foreign body or tympanic membrane perforation.]

5. **Any sore throat or fever?**

   [Patients with upper respiratory tract infection or pharyngitis may develop ear pain.]

6. **Have you noticed any odor from the ear?**

   [Consider a cholesteatoma from chronic middle ear infection.]

7. **Do you have any medical problems?**

   [Diabetics are at an increased risk for malignant otitis externa.]

8. **Are you taking any medications?**

   [Antineoplastic agents, certain antibiotics, salicylates, diuretics, and nonsteroidal anti-inflammatory drugs may all contribute to ear pain or hearing loss.]

9. **Any dizziness? Do you feel like you are moving or that the room is moving, as if you are drunk?**

   [Patients with labyrinthitis or a history of Ménière's disease may complain of ear pain.]

10. **Any discharge or fluid from the ear?**

    [In the early stages of otitis externa, there may be a green watery discharge that later becomes purulent and odor producing.]

11. **Did the pain improve after the discharge started?**

    [In acute otitis media with tympanic membrane rupture, patients may state that they improved after the onset of drainage.]

12. **Have you used any over the counter preparations?**

    [Consider salicylate toxicity.]

13. **Have you had this before?**

    [A common complication in patients with recurrent otitis media is cholesteatoma.]

14. **Does anything make the pain worse?**

    [In some cases of otitis externa, the pain is exacerbated by chewing.]

15. **Any nausea or vomiting associated with the pain?**

    [Vertigo, tinnitus, nausea, vomiting, and hearing loss suggest acute labyrinthitis.]

16. **Have you traveled recently by airplane?**

    [May contribute to sudden hearing loss secondary to cochlea rupture. Sudden hearing loss in the absence of barotraumas suggests vascular insufficiency.]

17. **Have you noticed any blisters on or around the ear?**

    [Vesicles or blisters on the auricle, in conjunction with severe pain, hearing loss, and vertigo, are seen with Ramsay-Hunt syndrome, also known as herpes zoster.]

18. **Have you had any itching of the ear?**

    [In otitis externa, itching progresses to severe inflammation, swelling, and discharge.]

19. **Any ringing in the ear?**

    [Consider tinnitus, Ménière's disease, or infection. Tinnitus may be the first symptom of acoustic schwannoma.]

20. **Was the hearing loss sudden? Is it one or both ears?**

    [Tinnitus may be the first symptom of acoustic schwannoma.]

21. **Has the child been pulling or tugging at the ear?**

    [In children, this may be the only sign of ear infection.]

DON'T FORGET TO ASK:

- Any history of hearing loss?
- History of associated vertigo or dizziness
- Presence of fever
- History of trauma or injury
- Hearing loss
- Recent swimming

EDEMA

1. **Do you have any significant past medical history?**

   [Most patients with noninflammatory generalized edema suffer from cardiac, renal, or hepatic disorders.]

2. **Have you had any shortness of breath or wheezing?**

   [Consider congestive heart failure.]

3. **Have you had fever?**

   [Local tenderness and increased temperature suggest inflammation.]

4. **Have you noticed the swelling in one place or is it all over?**

   [Localized edema may result from thrombophlebitis or chronic lymphangitis. Cardiac edema occurs symmetrically in the legs, pretibial region, and ankles.]

5. **Are you taking any medications?**

   [Ask about diuretics, thyroid medications, and antihypertensive medications.]

6. **Do you find that your jewelry or clothing is tighter?**

   [This is one of the earliest signs of edema and may be the first complaint of the patient.]

7. **Have you noticed any change in the size of your body?**

   [Ascites and a history of hepatic disease characterize edema of hepatic origin.]

8. **Do you notice the swelling mostly in the morning?**

[Edema that is associated with heart failure tends to be more extensive in the evening.]

9. **Any history of injury or trauma?**

[Consider fractures, sprains, and contusions.]

10. **Are you feeling pain over the swollen area?**

[Edema associated with heart failure or cardiac disease is generally not painful; consider trauma, arthritic processes, thrombophlebitis.]

11. **Do you smoke?**

[Cigarette smokers have an increased incidence of heart disease.]

12. **Have you had any breast or chest surgery?**

[Edema of one leg or of one or both arms is usually the result of venous or lymphatic obstruction.]

13. **How are things at home? Any new stresses, work, school, marriage, children?**

[Although rare, idiopathic edema, seen almost exclusively in women, often with psychosocial difficulties, will present with periodic episodes of edema.]

DON'T FORGET TO ASK:

- Significant past medical history
- Current medications
- History of shortness of breath

EPISTAXIS

In the elderly, the nasal mucosa can become very dry, and "rubbing" or "picking" can cause significant epistaxis.

1. Have you ever had this before? How often?

[Patients reporting a history of frequent epistaxis, without a history of trauma, may have a blood dyscrasia.]

2. Do you have any medical problems?

[Consider uncontrolled hypertension, bleeding diatheses, polycythemia vera, acute sinusitis, and, although rare, nasal angiomas or arterial venous malformations.]

3. Are you taking any medications?

[Particularly ask about aspirin, Coumadin/ heparin, vitamin E, or nonsteroidal anti- inflammatory drugs.]

4. Have you recently had a cold or "stuffy" nose?

[Minor epistaxis may occur in the course of infections of the upper respiratory tract.]

5. Do you have any significant family history?

[A family history of repeat hemorrhages may suggest Osler-Rendu-Weber syndrome.]

6. Have you recently traveled out of the country?

[Acute epistaxis may develop in typhoid fever or malaria.]

7. Any history of injury or trauma?

[This is important when ruling out the possibility of fractures.]

8. Have you been "picking" or rubbing your nose?

[The most common cause of epistaxis is "nose picking."]

9. **Have you seen the child put anything into the nose?**

[Foreign body is a frequent cause of epistaxis in children.]

DON'T FORGET TO ASK:

- Significant past medical history
- If the patient is taking medications
- History of injury or trauma
- Frequency of episodes

CHAPTER 17

EYE COMPLAINTS

Painless, sudden, and unilateral loss of vision, complete or incomplete, may result from central retinal artery occlusion.

1. **Do you have any changes in your vision? Any double vision?**

   [Dislocation the of lens may cause double vision or blurred vision. Also connective tissue disease like Marfan's syndrome.]

2. **Have you had any loss of vision?**

   [Amaurosis fugax and central vein occlusion can present with unilateral sudden loss of vision. Also consider central retinal artery occlusion.]

3. **Did this come on suddenly or gradually?**

   [Sudden painless visual loss is usually vascular; call ophthalmology quick!]

If vision loss is gradual, over several hours, central retinal vein occlusion or optic neuritis should be considered.

4. **Do you have any eye pain?**

   [Consider glaucoma; uritis is characterized by pain, photophobia, and lacrimation. Corneal infection, corneal erosion.]

5. **Any discharge or mucus from the eye?**

   [Bacterial conjunctivitis or corneal infection.]

6. **Any significant past medical history, like diabetes or hypertension?**

   [Patients with a long history of diabetes mellitus, or who are poorly controlled, are at increased risk for diabetic retinopathy blindness, glaucoma, or retinal detachment. Hypertensives also are at increased risk.]

Infection is the most common corneal disease.

7. **Any history of injury or trauma to the eye?**

   [Sudden loss of vision after a direct injury is consistent with retinal detachment. Also think of traumatic iritis, especially if the eye is infected.]

8. **Is there a sensation like something is being pulled over the eye like a shadow?**

   [Common complaint in retinal detachment.]

> In uritis the pain is in affected eye when light is directed into the opposite eye.

9. **Do you see flashing lights?**

   [Patients with uncontrolled diabetes are susceptible to retinal detachment and may complain of intermittent "flashing lights."]

10. **Do you see halos around lights?**

    [Cataracts or corneal edema. This symptom is also seen with acute angle-closure glaucoma.]

11. **If you cover one eye does the double vision stop?**

    [Binocular diplopia can be from mechanical restriction of the globe like in Graves' disease, trauma, myasthenia gravis.]

12. **Any history of recent eye surgery?**

    [Endophthalmitis commonly seen after eye surgery or trauma; patients have fever, pain, visual disturbances, and discharge.]

13. **Are the lids stuck together in the morning?**

    [Patients with bacterial conjunctivitis will complain of crusting of lids, particularly in the AM.]

14. **Have you noticed excessive tearing?**

    [Consider blocked nasolacrimal duct, congenital glaucoma, or, most commonly, irritation of the ocular surface.]

15. **Does the eye itch?**

    [Allergic conjunctivitis and viral conjunctivitis are associated with pruritus and clear discharge.]

16. **Do you feel like something is in the eye? Does blinking make it worse?**

    [Corneal impairment produces foreign body sensation exacerbated by blinking, like corneal abrasion.]

17. **Where is the pain located?**

    [Boring pain from the temporal region can be a sign of temporal arteritis or optic neuritis.]

18. Are your eyes sensitive to light?

[Uritis and keratitis, meningitis, migraine, subarachnoid hemorrhage. All can cause photophobia.]

19. Did you swallow anything? Are you taking any medication?

[Methanol and quinine are direct toxins to the retina and can cause blindness; Coumadin may also cause blindness.]

20. Any history of arthritis of recent onset?

[In suspected Reiter's syndrome, arthritis is acute and accompanied by fever and malaise and involves lower extremities.]

21. Have you had any urinary complaints? Urgency, frequency? Does it hurt to urinate? Any difficulty with the stream of urine?

[Urethritis followed by conjunctivitis and rheumatologic findings suggests Reiter's syndrome.]

22. Have you had any fever?

[Temporal arteritis can manifest with fever.]

23. Any nausea or vomiting or abdominal pain since or with the onset of eye pain?

[Glaucoma can present with nausea, vomiting, and abdominal pain.]

24. Have you had any recent eye surgery?

[Can indicate endophthalmitis.]

25. Have you had any recent sinus infection?

[Orbital cellulitis can be caused by direct extension of sinus infection.]

26. Any headache with or since the onset of eye pain?

[Consider glaucoma or migraine.]

27. Have you recently had any head injury?

[Forceful or blunt injury can cause hemorrhage or retinal detachment.]

28. **Did redness come on after straining or coughing?**

    [Rupture of a conjunctival blood vessel.]

29. **Did you have any pain, vesicles, or sensitivity around or near the eye before the onset of pain?**

    [Think of zoster.]

30. **If you look all the way to your left or right, can you see objects?**

    [Abnormalities of the intracranial visual pathway usually affect the peripheral visual field rather than the central field.]

31. **Does the eye hurt to move?**

    [As in orbital cellulitis.]

32. **Any history of genital herpes?**

    [Patients may infrequently infect themselves. If patient has a history of genital herpes, ask about touching the lesions or if they are using the same washcloth for body and face.]

DON'T FORGET TO ASK:

- Onset of symptoms
- Recent history of injury or trauma
- Vision loss
- Eye pain

FEVER

Malignant hyperthermia is characterized by a rapid rise in temperature in response to inhalation anesthetics.

1. How long have you had fever?

[Sudden onset almost always indicates infection, whereas long-term fever may indicate chronic potentially life-threatening pathology.]

2. Is the fever all the time or only during the day or night?

[Intermittent fever is characteristic in abscess, lymphoma, and tuberculosis.]

3. Have you had any cough or a cold?

[Consider upper respiratory tract infection.]

4. Any history of ear or throat pain or discomfort?

[Acute otitis media or pharyngitis often presents with fever.]

Intermittent fevers are characteristic in pyogenic infections like abscess or lymphoma.

5. Have you had any back pain?

[Nephrolithiasis or pyelonephritis, although pyelonephritis patients are quite toxic appearing.]

6. Do you have any pain in your belly?

[Consider cholecystitis, cholangitis, appendicitis, pelvic inflammatory disease, or splenic abscess.]

7. Any problems at all making urine? Does it hurt or burn? Are you going more than usual?

[Consider urinary tract infection, with episodes of ureteral obstruction due to stones or pyelonephritis.]

8. Do you have any medical problems?

[In chronic illness, patients may present with fever that is gradual in onset and steady.]

9. **Are you taking any medications? Any new medications?**

[Be sure to ask about new medications; patients may not always mention this.]

10. **Does it hurt to take a deep breath?**

[Pleuritic chest pain with fever may indicate pneumonia.]

11. **Have you recently traveled out of the country?**

[Consider malaria, typhoid, or tuberculosis.]

12. **Any diarrhea or constipation?**

[Consider viral or bacterial infection or appendicitis.]

13. **Do you feel hungry?**

[Also ask the patient if they feel hungry but cannot eat. Is the sensation of hunger present?]

14. **Any shortness of breath or difficulty breathing?**

[Consider pneumonia or bronchiectasis.]

15. **Have you recently had any procedures or operations?**

[Think of wound infection and, in rare instances, foreign body, uterine perforation, iatrogenic infection.]

16. **When was the last time that you had sex?**

[The incubation period for sexually transmitted pathogens may coincide with onset of fever.]

17. **Have you had any joint pain or discomfort?**

[Gout, chronic arthritis or rheumatoid disease, mononucleosis, or gonococcal disease.]

18. **Have you been in a wooded area lately, hiking, or gardening?**

[Insect bites, mosquitoes, ticks, spiders.]

19. **Have you noticed any change in mental status? (For elderly patients)**

[Acute onset of confusion with fever in the elderly may be the first signs of urinary tract infection.]

20. **Have you taken anything to relieve the fever? Did it help and how much have you taken?**

    [Relapsing or recurring fever not responding to analgesics indicates serious pathology. Consider abscess. Also, fever that is resistant to analgesics may indicate underdosing by the patient.]

21. **When was the last time that you took something?**

    [Always ask about self-medication, particularly aspirin, acetaminophen, nonsteroidal anti-inflammatory drugs, all of which may mask fever.]

22. **Have you had any abnormal vaginal discharge?**

    [Although some of the pathogens associated with pelvic inflammatory disease are asymptomatic like chlamydia, one sexually transmitted disease generally follows another.]

23. **Any significant weight loss?**

    [Fever of abrupt onset is associated with bacterial or viral infections like pharyngitis, upper respiratory tract infection, pneumonia, otitis media, to name a few.]

24. **Have you had any night sweats?**

    [Consider tuberculosis or human immunodeficiency virus infection.]

25. **Have you seen the child pulling or tugging at ears?**

    [May be the first indication of otitis in children.]

26. **Have you had any joint pain or discomfort?**

    [Gout, chronic arthritis or rheumatoid disease, mononucleosis, or gonococcal disease.]

DON'T FORGET TO ASK:

- History of upper respiratory tract infection symptoms
- Duration of fever and quality
- Presence of pain and location
- Has patient taken over the counter analgesics, when, and did it help?
- Significant past medical history

HEADACHE

The headache of meningitis or subarachnoid hemorrhage occurs usually in a single attack over a period of days.

1. **Where is the pain mostly?**

   [Cluster headaches are unilateral, and tension headaches are "band"-like and bilateral.]

2. **When did the pain start?**

   [Onset of headache after the age of 50 is suggestive; consider temporal arteritis or a mass lesion.]

3. **On a scale of 1 to 10, with 10 the worst, rate your pain.**

   [Simply put, the answer to this will indicate severity.]

Headache must be evaluated very carefully.

4. **Any history of nausea or vomiting?**

   [Consider migraine or space-occupying lesion.]

5. **Have you had fever?**

   [Meningitis may be a result of systemic infection. Also consider encephalitis, Lyme disease, and collagen vascular disease.]

6. **Any blurred vision?**

   [Consider migraine, carotid dissection, or temporal arteritis.]

Family, work, or social obligations can lead to greater stress and development of tension headaches.

7. **Do you feel like the room is moving or that you are moving?**

   [Dizziness or vertigo may be a finding with cerebral infarction, stroke, or migraine.]

8. **Is the pain constant or off and on?**

[Cluster headache is constant and may be unremitting. Constant pain with significant neurologic findings may indicate a bleed or space-occupying lesion. Temporal arteritis may also elicit constant pain.]

9. **Have you had this headache before?**

[Headaches caused by brain tumor are described as "new" or "different."]

10. **Did you take anything over the counter to make it better? Did it help?**

[Headache associated with brain tumor is resistant to analgesics.]

11. **Did the pain wake you?**

[Cluster headache may present as unilateral orbital pain occurring 2 to 3 hours after fully asleep; may occur nightly for a few weeks or months.]

12. **Are you taking any medications?**

[Pay special attention to history of oral contraceptive use or antihypertensive medication. Other drugs that may cause meningeal irritation are Tegretol and nonsteroidal anti-inflammatory drugs.]

13. **Do you smoke?**

[A history of smoking predisposes patient to hypertension and coronary artery disease and stroke.]

14. **Any medical problems?**

[Patients with a history of coronary artery disease or hypertension may be taking medications that exacerbate headache, like nitrates. Also ask about human immunodeficiency virus status.]

15. **What kind of work do you do?**

[Consider occupational or environmental exposure to carbon monoxide.]

16. **How are things at home?**

    [Family, work, or social obligations can lead to increased stress and development of tension headache.]

17. **Any history of fainting?**

    [A space-occupying lesion, subarachnoid hemorrhage, or carotid dissection may all cause syncope.]

18. **Have you noticed any "white lights" before your eyes?**

    [Patients with a history of migraines may complain of seeing "flashing lights."]

19. **Have you noticed any odor just before headache?**

    [Some migraines may be heralded by an aura.]

20. **Have you had any weakness in your hands or arms and legs?**

    [With a brain tumor, seizures, weakness, and subtle cognitive changes may be present.]

21. **Any history of recent trauma or injury?**

    [Consider subarachnoid hemorrhage or carotid dissection.]

22. **Where is the pain located on your head?**

    [The headache of subdural hematoma is often bitemporal; generalized cluster headache and trigeminal neuroglia are strictly unilateral. Migraine may be bifrontal, and tension headache is "band"-like and bilateral.]

23. **Any history of postnasal drip?**

    [Sinusitis, cluster headache.]

24. **Is pain worse when bending down?**

    [Patients with sinusitis may often complain that the headache pain is worse when bending forward. Headache associated with sinusitis is typically frontal.]

25. **Is pain more noticeable after falling asleep?**

[Cluster headache is constant, with associated unilateral orbital pain which occurs 2 to 3 hours after fully asleep. May occur nightly for a few weeks or months.]

26. **Did any thing or food precipitate the attack?**

[Coffee, ethyl alcohol, birth control pills, or sugar.]

27. **Any nausea or vomiting?**

[Migraines classically occur early morning and may last 1 to 2 days and may have associated nausea and vomiting.]

28. **Did the pain come on gradually or suddenly?**

[A sudden or very acute attack of headache pain that peaks in minutes with associated neurologic signs may indicate aneurysm.]

29. **What does your head feel like?**

["Pressing" or "tight" describes tension headache.]

30. **Have you noticed a change in your periods or leaking from your breasts?**

[Consider pituitary tumor.]

31. **Is the headache worse if you move your eyes?**

[When pain is severe and accentuated by eye movement, a systemic infection like meningitis should be considered.]

32. **Have you had any tearing from one eye during the headache?**

[Think of cluster headaches, migraine, or glaucoma.]

33. **Do you have any jaw pain when you open your mouth?**

[Temporomandibular joint syndrome or temporal arteritis.]

34. **Any history of muscle aches?**

[As with temporal arteritis.]

35. Is this your "worst" headache?

[Look out! When patients present with "worst headache of my life" it may signify hemorrhage.]

36. Is this headache like the ones you usually have?

[Severe unusual headaches of abrupt onset may signal hemorrhage.]

37. Are the headaches occurring more often?

[Suspect mass lesion, subdural hematoma.]

DON'T FORGET TO ASK:

- Duration, position, and quality of headache
- Associated symptoms of nausea, vomiting, or syncope
- Significant past medical history
- History of ethyl alcohol or drugs
- Prescribed medications
- Any aura preceding onset of symptoms?
- Is this worst headache ever?
- Associated vertigo or blurred vision
- Did headache wake you from sleep?

HEMATURIA

1. **When did you first notice the blood/bleeding?**

   [Hematuria that occurs mainly at the beginning or end of voiding may be prostatic or urethral.]

   Though not common, keep in mind Munchausen's syndrome.

2. **Does it hurt or burn when you urinate? Are you urinating more than usual?**

   [Recurrent bladder infection in the male with chronic bacterial prostatitis is very similar to that seen with recurrent cystitis in women.]

3. **Have you had any abdominal pain?**

   [Female patients with cystitis will often complain of suprapubic discomfort. Infarction of the renal artery may cause sudden sharp pain in the flank or upper abdomen.]

   In women, many times a urinary tract infection will present with a complaint of vaginal bleeding, but if you ask if blood is noticeable when wiping, patient will say yes, but not in panties.

4. **Any history of trauma, fighting, playing around, recent motor vehicle accident, or fall?**

   [Acute complete occlusion of the main renal artery may follow blunt trauma to the abdomen or back.]

5. **What color is your urine?**

   [In acute glomerulonephritis, gross hematuria is common and is described by the patient as "smoky," "coffee," or "cola" colored.]

6. **Any significant past medical history?**

   [Common causes of hematuria include nephrolithiasis, benign and malignant lesions, tuberculosis, prostatitis, sickle cell, systemic lupus erythematosus, hypertension, diabetes, and disorders of coagulation.]

   Remember, any woman of childbearing age should have pregnancy test, if high index.

7. **Are you taking any medications?**

   [Individuals who ingest large amounts of analgesics are prone to develop tubulointerstitial damage. Also consider anticoagulants.]

8. **When was your last period?**

   [Toward the end of the menstrual cycle, there may remain a persistent brownish/bloody discharge that may mimic a true hematuria. Be specific; ask the patient if menses are totally finished.]

9. **Have you recently had sore throat or upper respiratory tract infection?**

   [Although rare, acute poststreptococcal glomerulonephritis may follow the wake of pharyngeal or cutaneous infection. The onset of signs and symptoms is usually 6 to 10 days.]

10. **Have you noticed any bleeding after defecating?**

    [Consider hemorrhoids.]

11. **Have you recently had any surgical procedures?**

    [Consider iatrogenic damage to the urethra or Foley catheter insertion.]

DON'T FORGET TO ASK:

- History of dysuria, urgency, or frequency
- History of fever
- Abdominal or back pain
- History of trauma or injury
- Medication history
- Significant past medical history

JOINT PAIN

1. **How long have you had this?**

   [The length of time that the patient has had the signs and symptoms alters diagnostic considerations.]

2. **Did the pain come on suddenly or gradually?**

   [In rheumatoid arthritis, the symptoms appear gradually. In infectious processes or gout, the onset is usually more acute. Osteoarthritis and fibrositis may have a more indolent presentation.]

3. **Have you had fever?**

   [Consider rheumatoid arthritis or systemic lupus erythematosus. In infectious arthritis, the onset is usually acute. Fever and joint pain may also be associated with acute pharyngitis/tonsillitis, flu, or upper respiratory tract infection.]

4. **Do you have any significant family history or past medical history?**

   [Patients with past medical history or family history of diabetes, collagen vascular disease, sickle cell, or arthritis may complain of joint pain.]

5. **Are you taking any medications, including supplements or herbal preparations? How much and which medications?**

   [Remember, signs and symptoms may be decreased in patients receiving corticosteroids, or immunosuppressive drugs. Always ask patients if they have taken any over the counter nonsteroidal anti-inflammatory drugs.]

6. **What were you doing when you noticed the pain?**

   [This is important when ascertaining exacerbating factors.]

7. **Do you have pain in all your joints or just in one particular area?**

   [Rheumatoid arthritis tends to be symmetric, whereas the spondyloarthropathies are asymmetric. In ankylosing spondylitis, the initial symptom may be low back pain without history of trauma with associated pain of hips, buttocks, and shoulders.]

8. **Have you noticed the pain in other places?**

   [Disorders such as polymyositis and fibrositis involve more than a single site.]

9. **What kind of work do you do? Have you recently started a fitness program?**

   [Consider muscle or joint strain associated with strength training. Pain aggravated by movement is also common in rheumatoid arthritis.]

10. **Does the pain improve as the day progresses?**

    [In rheumatoid arthritis, patients may complain of generalized stiffness that is most pronounced after periods of inactivity; morning stiffness is a hallmark of rheumatoid arthritis.]

11. **Does anything make the pain better or worse? What?**

    [In degenerative joint disease, the pain is improved while at rest.]

12. **Have you noticed any redness or discoloration to the area?**

    [Consider infectious arthritis, gout, or trauma.]

13. **Any history of injury or trauma?**

    [Trauma or gout are typically focal, involving a single site.]

14. **Does it hurt to touch the area?**

    [Patients with suspected gout will have an extremely painful, erythematous, often edematous focal area. Also consider a septic joint or arthritis.]

15. **When was the last time that you had sex? Did you use a condom?**

    [Especially in young people or those sexually active with multiple sex partners, consider joint pain associated with gonococcus.]

16. **Have you had any penile discharge that you did not have checked out?**

    [Again, consider septic joint associated with gonococcus.]

17. **Have you had any long-standing problems with your sight or frequent gastrointestinal complaints?**

    [This suggests orthostatic hypertension, which may be related to cardiac medications, exercise, or volume depletion.]

DON'T FORGET TO ASK:

- Onset and duration of symptoms
- Significant past medical history
- History of fever
- Medication history
- What makes pain better or worse?

LACERATIONS AND ABRASIONS

1. **What were you doing when this happened?**

   [It is important to identify conditions that place the patient at risk for infection and possible foreign body.]

2. **Do you have any medical problems?**

   [Diabetes, chronic renal failure, and use of steroids increase wound infection rate. Elderly patients are at higher risk of poor tissue healing. Also, chronic alcoholism and patients with advanced liver disease may have poor wound healing.]

3. **Do you have any allergies?**

   [In addition to antibiotic allergy, it is important to ask about possible allergy to latex or Betadine.]

4. **When did this happen? How long ago?**

   [There is really no *"golden hour"* for laceration repair. However, generally speaking, if the wound is more than 8 hours old and is particularly "dirty," closure is not recommended. Copious irrigation and topical or systemic antibiotic therapy may suffice.]

5. **When was your last tetanus shot?**

   [If tetanus immunization was more than 5 years ago, a standard booster dose of tetanus-diphtheria should be given.]

6. **What cut you?**

   [The type of force applied at the time of injury predicts the likelihood of infection. Crush injuries are more susceptible to infection than are wounds resulting from the more shearing forces that are commonly seen in the Emergency Department.]

7. **Are you taking any medications?**

[Particularly anticoagulants, nonsteroidal anti-inflammatory drugs, aspirin, or vitamin E, all of which may prolong bleeding. Corticosteroids suppress wound contraction and decrease wound re-epithelialization. Chemotherapeutic agents arrest cell production and reduce protein synthesis.]

8. **Did you try to remove any dirt or foreign body at home?**

[This may increase the likelihood of incidence of infection.]

9. **What is your human immunodeficiency virus status?**

[Self-explanatory. Do not be embarrassed to ask the patient. Know your population.]

10. **Did anything fall on you?**

[Don't forget to get x-rays in suspected crush injuries to rule out an open fracture.]

11. **Have you had any limitation of movement in the area involving the injury?**

[Always check for damage to deep or superficial tendons.]

12. **What was the bleeding like before you wrapped it?**

[A description of *"pumping"* or *"shooting"* may indicate a more serious wound with arterial involvement.]

DON'T FORGET TO ASK:

- History of allergies
- Past medical history
- Is the patient taking medications?
- Mechanism of injury

MOTOR VEHICLE ACCIDENT

Loss of consciousness
warrants a head
computed tomography!

1. **When did this happen?**

   [The length of time between the accident and the time that the patient presents to the Emergency Department may be significant and will assist you in determining severity of symptoms.]

2. **Was there any loss of consciousness?**

   [Loss of consciousness after a motor vehicle accident warrants an in-depth neurologic evaluation.]

3. **Did you get out of the car at the scene of the accident?**

   [If the patient was ambulatory at the scene, major injury to C-spine or vertebrae can basically be ruled out.]

4. **Were you wearing a seat belt?**

   [Seatbelt injuries to the neck and upper chest can cause significant discomfort to the patient and in many cases considerable injury to the neck and chest. Check for carotid bruits.]

5. **Did you hit your head or chest?**

   [This is important when ruling out head injury or contusion of cardiac or visceral structures.]

6. **Did the air bags open?**

   [Air bag deployment can cause serious injuries, including superficial abrasions to face, neck, and forearms. In addition, many patients are allergic to the chemicals that are released at the time of deployment and may complain of cough or wheezing.]

7. **Are you having any headache, blurred vision, or dizziness?**

[These symptoms may be direct result of head injury, reaction to air bag chemicals, or the anxiety and stress associated with the accident.]

8. **Are you having any abdominal pain?**

[Careful physical examination will rule out injury to intra-abdominal structures like spleen, liver, or pancreas.]

9. **Have you had any back pain?**

[Rule out injury to vertebrae or retroperitoneal structures.]

10. **Have you had any urinary or bowel dysfunction?**

[This may indicate injury to sacral root and warrants further neurologic workup.]

11. **Have you had any shortness of breath or pain when you take a deep breath?**

[These symptoms may indicate rib fractures, pneumothorax or hemothorax.]

DON'T FORGET TO ASK:

- History of loss of consciousness
- Abdominal or back pain
- Urinary or bowel dysfunction

NAUSEA AND VOMITING

> If it walks like a duck and quacks like a duck, be careful: It may be a chicken.

1. **Have you had any fever?**

   [Systemic infections may initially present with nausea, vomiting, and fever. Possibility of viral hepatitis, appendicitis, peptic ulcer disease, cholecystitis.]

2. **Any abdominal pain?**

   [In acute appendicitis, nausea and vomiting develop after the onset of pain. Also think of acute cholecystitis, intestinal obstruction, pancreatitis, or, in the more critically ill patient, peritonitis.]

> No assumptions. Remember, your patient may not present like the textbook.

3. **Have you had any symptoms of cough or runny nose?**

   [Consider an upper respiratory infection or viral syndrome.]

4. **When was your last period?**

   [Always consider pregnancy and hyperemesis, which may be excessive with twin gestation and is rare after 12 weeks.]

5. **Have you had any diarrhea or constipation that is out of the ordinary?**

   [Consider food poisoning, particularly salmonella or shigella. Keep in mind appendicitis, pelvic inflammatory disease, or intestinal obstruction.]

> Try to rule out the obvious first.

6. **What color is the vomit?**

   [If the vomit contains free hydrochloric acid, this may be indicative of peptic ulcer. Blood indicates bleeding from the esophagus, stomach, or duodenum. In severe obstruction, vomit becomes yellowish to feculent.]

7. **Are you taking any medications to alleviate symptoms? Did they help?**

   [Symptoms of nausea and vomiting not relieved by over the counter preparations may indicate more serious pathology, especially in the presence of abdominal pain.]

Do not forget to get a pregnancy test in all women of childbearing age. *No matter what they say!*

8. **Have you had any abdominal surgery?**

   [Patients with a history of frequent or recent abdominal surgery may present with nausea and vomiting associated with intestinal obstruction.]

9. **What have you eaten over the last 48 hours?**

   [Consider endotoxins from food poisoning.]

10. **Does vomiting alleviate any abdominal discomfort that you might have?**

    [Vomiting may relieve the pain associated with peptic ulcer disease.]

11. **Are you taking any medications for other problems?**

    [Nonsteroidal anti-inflammatory drugs, oral contraceptives, and many antibiotics can cause episodes of nausea and vomiting. A large number of medications can cause the symptoms of nausea and vomiting.]

12. **What other medical problems do you have?**

    [Consider diabetic ketoacidosis, adrenal insufficiency, or hepatitis.]

13. **Have you noticed any change in size of your belly?**

    [Abdominal distention is classic in obstruction. Also think of ovarian cancer, Meigs' syndrome, or liver disease.]

14. **Does the nausea occur at any particular time? Is it worse after eating or better?**

    [Symptoms that are relieved by food suggest duodenal ulcer.]

15. Have you noticed any eye pain since the onset of nausea and vomiting?

[Acute angle-closure glaucoma may give rise to symptoms of nausea, vomiting, and abdominal pain.]

16. Any ringing in the ear? Or ear pain?

[Consider disorders like labyrinthitis or Ménière's disease.]

17. Have you been out of the country lately?

[Consider tainted food or water.]

18. Have you had dizziness or fainting?

[This may be an indication of volume depletion secondary to vomiting.]

19. How many times have you vomited?

[Frequent vomiting may lead to secondary volume depletion. Consider the rest of your patient's history: persistent and severe vomiting is characteristic of obstruction.]

DON'T FORGET TO ASK:

- About possibility of pregnancy
- Symptoms of pain or fever
- Significant past medical history
- Duration and quality of vomiting
- Dizziness

NEEDLESTICK

1. **What were you doing when this happened?**

   [This is important when considering antibiotic coverage, tetanus, or human immunodeficiency virus counseling.]

2. **When was your last tetanus shot?**

   [If tetanus immunization was more than 5 years before injury, a standard booster dose of tetanus should be given.]

3. **Do you have any allergies?**

   [Important when considering antibiotic coverage.]

4. **Have you ever been immunized for hepatitis?**

   [This is important when determining risk for development of hepatitis. It also establishes a baseline.]

5. **Do you know the history of the patient?**

   [This is important in determining the degree of risk for developing human immunodeficiency virus, hepatitis, or wound infection.]

6. **What is your human immunodeficiency virus status and when were you last tested?**

   [Again, this is important to establish a baseline.]

DON'T FORGET TO ASK:

- Mechanism of injury
- History of the patient
- History of allergies
- Tetanus immunization

ORAL COMPLAINTS, TEETH, AND GINGIVA

Lead poisoning and bismuth poisoning may be manifested by a dark line along the gingival margin.

1. **Have you had pain or difficulty swallowing, any drooling or difficulty holding saliva in the mouth?**

   [Consider peritonsillar abscess and call an ear, nose, and throat specialist!]

2. **Any history of fever?**

   [Acute tonsillitis or pharyngitis, herpes simplex type 1, mononucleosis. All can cause fever.]

3. **Have you had this before?**

   [In herpes labialis, patients may have a prodrome of tingling, then pain and a history of previous eruption.]

4. **Do you have any significant past medical history? Do you have any medical problems for which a doctor is treating you?**

   [Fishy odor to the breath is found in patients with hepatic failure.]

5. **Does your tongue and/or gums hurt?**

   [Patients with Vincent's angina present with the acute onset of gingival pain that is worsened by spicy foods and accompanied by bleeding, fetid odor, and taste alteration.]

6. **Have you had a particularly foul odor from the mouth?**

   [Consider stomatitis, abscess, or severe periodontal disease.]

7. **Are you a smoker?**

   [Persistent laryngitis, pharyngitis, and pain in a patient who smokes may indicate malignancy.]

8. **Have you noticed any sores on the gums, tongue, or inside the mouth?**

   [Think of herpes, hand-foot-mouth disease, primary or tertiary syphilis, Stevens-Johnson syndrome, candida, and neoplastic disease. Extensive ulcerations of the gingiva, buccal mucosa, lips, soft palate, pharynx, and/or tonsils may occur in agranulocytosis. In Plummer-Vinson syndrome, the tongue is red, smooth, and sore and the patient may have difficulty swallowing.]

9. **Have you had abnormal bleeding from the gums?**

   [This may signify gingivitis or one of the leukemias, particularly monocytic leukemia.]

10. **Have you noticed any redness or change in the texture of the tongue?**

    [Consider vitamin B_{12} deficiency/pernicious anemia.]

11. **Any discoloration to the gums or inside of the mouth?**

    [Heavy metal pigmentation, drug ingestion, bluish-black spots as is seen in Addison's disease. Dark brown spots on lips, buccal mucosa, and palate in Peutz-Jeghers syndrome, or petechiae and ulceration which can be seen in leukemia.]

12. **Any burning of the tongue or mouth?**

    [Vitamin B deficiency may give rise to reddening and ulceration of the oral mucosa and tongue, with occasional complaint of burning of the tongue and fissuring at the corner of the lips.]

13. **Have you felt particularly tired or like you have the flu?**

    [Mononucleosis will give rise to fatigue, sore throat malaise, low grade fever, and enlarged cervical nodes.]

14. Have you any history of anemia?

[Particularly pernicious anemia, in which you may see ulceration xerostomia and infection.]

15. Does eating make the gum pain worse?

[In sialolithiasis the pain in salivary gland is worse with or after eating.]

16. Have you had any swelling of the floor of the mouth?

[In Ludwig's angina, patients may report swelling of the floor of the mouth and difficulty swallowing saliva.]

DON'T FORGET TO ASK:

- Duration of symptoms
- Significant past medical history
- History of fever
- Drooling
- History of smoking

RASH

1. **Does it hurt?**

   [Consider herpes zoster.]

2. **Does it itch?**

   [All of the following may be pruritic: chicken pox, insect bite, contact dermatitis, or connective tissue disorder.]

3. **Did you notice any tingling or sensitivity before the onset of the rash?**

   [Herpes zoster often presents with a prodrome of skin sensitivity and tingling of the affected area.]

4. **Any history of fever?**

   [Consider communicable diseases in children, Rocky Mountain spotted fever, herpes zoster, meningitis, toxic shock syndrome, or scarlet or rheumatic fever.]

5. **Have you had any body aches or joint pain?**

   [Complication of streptococcal infection.]

6. **Do you have any long-standing medical problems?**

   [Consider diabetes mellitus, immunocompromised patients, and patients with renal disease.]

7. **Are you taking any new medications?**

   [Be sure to also ask if there has been any change in medication.]

8. **Are you allergic to any foods or medications?**

   [Consider adverse reactions or side effects from medication.]

> In women of childbearing age, ask about tampon use.

79

9. Have you eaten anything that you have never tried before?

[Food allergen.]

10. Have you used any perfumes, powders, lotions, or creams?

[Also ask about hair spray, hair dye, new linen or clothes.]

11. Any sore throat?

[Consider communicable diseases, hand-foot-mouth disease, Rocky Mountain spotted fever, and scarlet fever.]

12. Did the rash always look like this or did it look different when it first began?

[The patient may not present to the Emergency Department at initial onset and may have partially self-medicated at home. By the time the patient arrives at the Emergency Department, the rash may have changed in appearance.]

13. At any point did you notice blisters?

[Consider chicken pox, herpes zoster, impetigo, allergic reaction, bacterial or fungal infection, or sun sensitivity.]

14. Did the rash come on suddenly or gradually?

[With contact dermatitis or food or medication allergy, the rash may develop suddenly, whereas patients with long-standing systemic disease may have a more gradual onset.]

15. Have you been working in the yard or a wooded area?

[Consider poison ivy, oak, or sumac. Keep in mind spider bites, tick bites, or fungal infections.]

16. What kind of work do you do?

[Patient may be exposed to an allergen that is present in the workplace.]

17. **Where did the rash start?**

[In children, if the rash began on the face or trunk, consider communicable diseases, Rocky Mountain spotted fever, or prickly heat. Erythema multiforme begins on the palms, soles, arms, and legs. Rash appearing on the cheeks in a "butterfly" appearance may indicate lupus erythematosus. Rashes that begin in the inter-trigenous areas may indicate scabies.]

DON'T FORGET TO ASK:

- Any history of fever
- History of pain
- Onset of symptoms
- Associated symptoms like sore throat, joint pain, or headache

SEIZURES, FAINTING, AND LOSS OF CONSCIOUSNESS

If all the laboratory values look "great" but your patient looks ill, you had better look again!

1. **Has this ever happened to you before?**

   [It is important to explore whether similar events have occurred. This may help identify seizure disorder or vasovagal event.]

2. **What were you doing when you fainted or had the seizure?**

   [The answer to this question may assist in ruling out cardiac versus other precipitating factors, such as, was the patient urinating or engaged in a sports activity.]

The most common cause of new onset seizure in the elderly is stroke.

3. **Was anyone with you when this happened? Did anyone witness the episode?**

   [Seizure patients may experience a period of postictal confusion and lethargy that may last for hours and they may not remember the event. Witnesses should be asked about loss of consciousness, incontinence, and if there was tonic clonic activity.]

4. **Have you had headache just before the episode or have you had headaches in the past that were not your usual headache?**

   [Severe headaches may suggest a subarachnoid hemorrhage.]

Eclampsia should be considered in the seizing pregnant patient who is more than 20 weeks' pregnant.

5. **Have you recently had fever?**

   [Identify seizure precipitants, including systemic infection or new anatomic lesions, that may be suspected in patients with malignancy.]

6. **Any history of chest pain?**

   [The answer to this question will assist in iden-
   tifying a cardiac cause of loss of consciousness.
   Ask about a history of palpitations or dysrhyth-
   mias. Syncope secondary to dysrhythmia
   carries the highest 1-year mortality and 24%
   of incidence of sudden death.]

7. **Did you smell or taste anything "funny" before
   the episode?**

   [Unusual aromas may represent seizure activity; this is referred to as an aura.]

8. **Any recent injury to the head or chest? A fall or
   car accident?**

   [Past history of trauma or head injury may
   suggest a seizure cause.]

9. **Are you taking any medications, over the
   counter or prescribed by a doctor?**

   [Most culpable are digitalis, alpha-methyldopa,
   and propanolol, although there are a vast number of medications that may cause syncope,
   seizures, and loss of consciousness. Among
   these are psychotropic drugs. Also, ask about
   new medications or changes in dosing.]

10. **Do you have any medical problems?**

    [A history of transient ischemic attacks, cere-
    brovascular accidents, diabetes mellitus, hyper-
    tension, and cardiac disease, including the
    presence of a pacemaker, may be a seizure
    precipitant.]

11. **When was your last period? Was it normal
    for you?**

    [Always rule out pregnancy as a cause of syn-
    cope in women of childbearing age.]

12. **Did you have any abdominal pain or back pain
    before the episode?**

    [Consider perforated viscus, hemoperitoneum,
    ectopic pregnancy, or ruptured aneurysm.]

13. Do you have heavy periods?

[Menorrhagia may result in secondary anemia, predisposing the patient to syncope.]

14. Do you have any allergies?

[An occult allergen may be a precipitant of syncope or seizure.]

15. How is your appetite?

[Unfortunately, more and more young women are developing eating disorders. Simple hypoglycemia may lead to syncope.]

16. Did you come around right away or did it take some time?

[Epileptic seizures usually last less than 2 minutes and are followed by a postictal period. Vasovagal syncope is brief, with recovery minutes after assuming a prone position.]

17. Did you urinate or defecate on yourself at the time of the episode?

[Patients with motor seizures frequently have fecal or urinary incontinence.]

18. Did you have any feeling that your heart was beating too fast or skipping beats before this?

[Think of vasovagal episode or palpitations, which may be secondary to anxiety.]

19. Have you noticed any change in the color of your stool? Is it black?

[Patients may have an unreported history of "dark stools" which can lead to anemia and secondary syncope.]

20. Were you standing or sitting when you had this episode?

[A syncopal episode generally occurs while the patient is awake and is positionally elevated. Seizures can occur at any time with the patient in any position. The patient may be asleep or lying flat.]

21. **Have you used any street drugs like cocaine, "special K," or heroin? Are you sniffing prescribed medications like OxyContin, Ritalin, or Lortab?**

[Many patients, particularly teens, are sniffing controlled substances. The most common today are Ritalin and OxyContin.]

22. **Were you on the toilet when the episode occurred?**

["Straining" during constipation may precipitate a vasovagal episode.]

DON'T FORGET TO ASK:

- Prior history of this event
- Significant past medical history
- Always consider pregnancy
- Aura before episode?

SEXUAL ASSAULT

This is a very sensitive subject. Patience and understanding are very important.

1. **When did this happen? What time?**

   [Duration of time between incident and presentation to Emergency Room will determine if specimens will be obtainable. Sperm can remain in cervical mucus for as long as 10 days.]

2. **Were you alone?**

   [This becomes important in the case where witnesses are needed]

3. **Do you know where you were when this happened?**

   [This question will also help establish if the patient is oriented.]

Allow your patient the time to tell *you* the story.

4. **Were you hit, punched, or slapped?**

   [Possible head, ear, or eye injury. This also becomes important when obtaining specimens for the "Vitullo Kit."]

5. **Did you fight back?**

   [Material for DNA analysis may be found under the fingernails.]

Give the patient back some control; involve them in as much of the examination as they are willing.

6. **How many people attacked you?**

   [Important in semen evaluation and DNA testing.]

7. **Was there any other kind of sex aside from sex in the vagina? Was there any sex in the rectum or oral sex?**

   [If the patient reports anal and oral sex, specimens for evidence should be taken from these areas.]

8. **Do you know if there was ejaculation inside of you? Did you feel wet after?**

[The patient may state that they are unsure of ejaculation, so to ask if they feel "wet" after the attack can assist in determining if there was ejaculation.]

> Be gentle with the speculum. Remember the patient was already violated once.

9. **Were there any objects used during the attack? Was anything else put into your vagina or rectum?**

[Blunt or sharp objects used during sexual assault may cause significant tissue trauma.]

10. **Are these the clothes that you were wearing? Are these the same underwear?**

[Body fluids like blood or semen may be found on clothes.]

> Police should *not* be in the examination room during history and physical.

11. **Have you bathed since the attack?**

[Bathing may have removed important evidence.]

12. **Have you brushed your teeth, eaten, or drank anything since the attack?**

[Again, this is important, because it may hinder specimen collection.]

> Reach for your empathy.

13. **Have you urinated or defecated?**

[Which may interfere with specimen collection.]

14. **When was your last period?**

[Pregnancy should be ruled out before starting antibiotic or oral contraceptives or possible x-rays.]

15. **Have you had any bleeding from the rectum or vagina since the attack?**

[Rule out tissue trauma.]

16. **Are you having any abdominal pain?**

[Particularly during physically violent attacks, patients may sustain significant intra-abdominal injury.]

In suspected assault in children, ask if there are older children in the household.

17. Was there any ejaculation into the mouth?

[Specimens for Vitullo Kit should be taken from the mouth if the patient reports ejaculation into the mouth.]

18. At any time during the attack did you pass out?

[Rule out significant head injury.]

19. Were you forced to eat or drink anything?

[This may determine if toxicology screen is warranted.]

20. Are you taking medication?

[Including oral contraceptives.]

Let the patient know at the beginning of your history that some of the questions will be graphic.

21. Do you have any allergies?

[This will become important upon discharge when antibiotic prophylaxis for sexually transmitted disease is indicated.]

22. Have you had or been immunized for hepatitis? Or have you ever had syphilis?

[This establishes a base line for testing and treatment.]

Always do a hepatitis screen and rapid plasma reagent.

23. When was the last time that you had sex before this attack?

[Again, DNA analysis will be important here.]

Suspected Assault on Children

24. Have you noticed any unusual stains in the child's underwear?

[Which may be semen, blood or abnormal discharge.]

25. Has there been a remarkable change in the child's behavior, such as reclusiveness, decreased appetite, or violent/aggressive behavior?

[Although children may not always inform parents or adults of being sexually assaulted, their behavior may become very different from what is "normal." They may "act out."]

26. **Have teachers noticed a change in the child or reported a change in grades?**

    [Again, subtle behavior changes or drastic changes in school performance may indicate a problem.]

> In children, a tip off might be the child's obvious willingness to allow genital examination.

27. **Is the child "acting out" sexually? More than what is normal for children?**

28. **Have you noticed that the child is afraid or is reluctant to go to a familiar friend or family member?**

29. **Has the child complained of pain in the vagina or rectum?**

> If child is being left alone at home, ask about older siblings or adults in the household.

DON'T FORGET TO ASK:

- When was last menstrual period?
- When the patient was last sexually active before the attack
- About drinking, bathing, brushing teeth, urinating, defecating, or changing clothes since the attack
- About any history of loss of consciousness during or since the attack

SEXUALLY TRANSMITTED DISEASES

This is a very sensitive subject. Do not assume anything about your patient.

1. When did the symptoms begin?

[The incubation period of the various sexually transmitted diseases (STDs) will aid in diagnosis, and incubation period is very important in determining organism.]

2. When was the last time that you had sex?

[The incubation period and onset of symptoms are directly correlated with last sexual contact.]

3. Did you use protection? What type?

[Condoms are the most reliable form of contraception to protect against most sexually transmitted diseases. Other forms of spermicidals are not effective at all.]

Do not be ashamed to ask your patient if they were sexually active while on vacation.

4. Does it hurt or burn when you urinate? Are you going more than usual?

[Patients complaining of dysuria, urgency, and frequency may have a urinary tract infection related to chlamydia.]

5. Have you had any penile/vaginal discharge? What color?

[Remember that chlamydia may be asymptomatic in men and women. Always think of chlamydia and gonorrhea as traveling together. Thick greenish/yellow penile discharge is strongly indicative of gonorrhea, with *Trichomonas*; vaginal discharge is copious, greenish/yellow, and frothy.]

Stay culturally sensitive. Remember we live in a wonderfully diverse world.

6. Does discharge have any odor?

[A "fishy" or foul smell to vaginal discharge is indicative of bacterial vaginosis or foreign body.]

7. **Have you had any painful sores or blisters? Have you noticed any sores at all?**

   [Painful lesions are indicative of genital herpes. Also consider primary syphilis if lesions are painless.]

8. **Have you had itching?**

   [As with genital herpes or candida.]

9. **Did you notice any sensitivity or tingling before the onset of rash?**

   [This may herald the onset of genital herpes.]

10. **Do you have any pain in the groin?**

    [In lymphogranuloma, inguinal, penile, vulvar, and anal infection can lead to inguinal and femoral lymphadenitis.]

11. **Any pain in the testicles?**

    [Patients with orchitis or epididymitis complain of testicular pain.]

12. **Any abdominal pain?**

    [In women, consider onset of salpingitis.]

13. **Have you had anal sex?**

    [Cultures should be taken vaginally, rectally, and from the urethra.]

14. **Any pain or discharge from rectum?**

    [In anal gonorrhea, patients will complain of pain that increases with defecation.]

15. **How many partners do you have? All same sex?**

    [STDs are rare in strictly lesbian women and are increased in heterosexuals and gay men with multiple partners.]

16. **Have you had oral sex?**

    [Examine the tongue and posterior pharynx for lesions.]

17. **Have you noticed a clear "mucus"-like discharge from your penis?**

[This may be the only sign of chlamydia infection in men; in fact, many men will think this is semen.]

18. **Any history of fever?**

[Salpingitis, orchitis, epididymitis; all these patients may complain of fever.]

19. **Have you had any joint pain?**

[Patients with disseminated gonorrhea may complain of a painful, erythematous, warm joint.]

20. **Have you ever had a venereal disease before? Were you treated? Was your partner?**

[If there is a recent history of STD and the partner was not treated, reinfection must be considered.]

DON'T FORGET TO ASK:

- Last sexually active
- Was a condom used?
- Fever
- Abdominal or testicular pain
- When was last menstrual period?
- If patient is homosexual or heterosexual
- About penile or abnormal vaginal discharge

SHOULDER PAIN

1. What were you doing when this happened?

[Acromioclavicular joint dislocation is usually associated with contact sports, motor vehicle accidents, and falls. Clavicle fractures, which are most common in children, are usually caused by a lateral blow from a tackle, fall, or motor vehicle accident. Fractures that involve the proximal humerus occur typically in older patients and are usually the result of a fall onto an outstretched arm.]

2. Did the pain come on suddenly?

[Acute rotator cuff tears present with sudden, sharp, tearing pain, which may radiate down the arm to the elbow.]

3. How long have you had the pain?

[Chronic pain may be the result of acute injury or prolonged repetitive movement. The most common cause of chronic shoulder pain is rotator cuff tendonitis, which is common in patients who throw or swim.]

4. Any significant past medical history?

[Be sure that the pain is originating from the shoulder. You should always rule out other possibly life-threatening causes for shoulder pain, like a cardiac or gastrointestinal history. If there is no history of injury or trauma, you must look for other causes for shoulder pain. Adhesive capsulitis is often associated with diabetes or hypothyroidism.]

5. **Did the pain start somewhere else and then go to the shoulder?**

[Consider C-spine disorder, thoracic outlet syndrome, acute myocardial infarction, diaphragmatic irritation, diseases of the stomach, gallbladder, or pancreas.]

6. **Where is the pain mostly located?**

[Patients with pain caused by rotator cuff tendonitis often will place a hand over the lateral shoulder. Those with a clavicle fracture can point to the exact location with one finger.]

7. **When was your last period?**

[Always rule out pregnancy on all young women of childbearing age to rule out the possibility of ectopic pregnancy.]

8. **Have you had any abdominal pain?**

[Take the rest of your history into consideration. Consider the possibility of perforation, hemoperitoneum, free air, or foreign body.]

9. **Have you had any shortness of breath or difficulty breathing?**

[Injuries to the proximal third of the clavicle are caused by a direct blow to the anterior chest and can be associated with significant intrathoracic injury. Scapular fractures are highly associated with injuries to the ipsilateral lung, chest wall, and shoulder girdle.]

10. **Did the pain start with the shoulder?**

[Pain originating in the shoulder does not usually radiate past the elbow.]

11. **How did you fall?**

[Glenohumeral dislocation is usually caused by a fall on an abducted externally rotated arm.]

12. **Does any particular activity make the pain worse?**

[Patients who have rotator cuff disorder may complain of increased pain during movement of reaching forward or overhead.]

13. Is the pain worse at night?

[Painful arc syndrome is associated with chronic tendonitis. There is usually no history of trauma.]

14. Have you had this before?

[Posterior shoulder dislocations are rare and can be caused by significant trauma or seizure. These may be chronic or recurrent.]

15. Is the pain only in one shoulder?

[One or both shoulders may be involved with tendonitis of the shoulder.]

16. Do you have difficulty lifting your hand?

[Consider subscapularis injury if the patient cannot lift the hand.]

17. Any history of bursitis?

[Patients who have a long history of shoulder pain, secondary to rotator cuff tendonitis or bursitis, can be subject to chronic tearing of the rotator cuff muscles. These patients usually have a history of performing strenuous repetitive movements with the arms over the head.]

DON'T FORGET TO ASK:

- Significant past medical history
- Mechanism of injury
- Duration of symptoms
- Associated symptoms of shortness of breath
- History of abdominal pain
- History of chest pain

SINUSITIS

1. How long have you had the symptoms?

[Patients that have documented recurrences of sinusitis may have chronic sinusitis. Also, rule out allergens.]

2. Any history of fever?

[The diagnosis of acute purulent sinusitis is usually made when symptoms of fever, chills, pain, and tenderness occur in the involved sinus.]

3. Do you have a headache? Where?

[Frontal sinusitis is characterized by pain over the eyebrows.]

4. Have you recently had a cold or flu?

[The most common predisposing factor for development of sinusitis is upper respiratory tract infection.]

5. Have you had this before?

[A neoplastic lesion should be ruled out in patients who experience repeated episodes of acute sinusitis or with chronic symptoms and epistaxis.]

6. Are the headaches made worse by any particular position?

[In purulent sinusitis, patients may have recurrent frontal headaches that change in intensity with positions and disappear shortly after getting out of bed.]

7. Have you recently had any dental procedures?

[Gingivitis with abscesses of the roots of the upper bicuspid or molar teeth may predispose to sinusitis.]

8. **Are you taking any other medications?**

   [You may suspect other organisms in patients who are taking immunosuppressive drugs or antibiotics.]

9. **Did the antibiotics help?**

   [A nonobstructing lesion should be considered in recurrent episodes of sinusitis that do not respond to antibiotic therapy or fail traditional treatment.]

10. **Have you recently been swimming or diving?**

    [May predispose patient to sinusitis, especially lake swimming.]

11. **Any history of recent injury or trauma?**

    [Fractures of the sinus bones, especially frontal and ethmoid, may lead to infection.]

12. **Have you had pain in the teeth?**

    [With severe sinus infection, pain may be referred to the teeth.]

13. **Have you had recent onset of fever?**

    [Although rare, in patients with acute frontal sinusitis, the onset of a fever suggests possibility of subdural abscess.]

14. **Has the inside of your nose felt puffy or swollen?**

    [This may indicate nasal polyps.]

DON'T FORGET TO ASK:

- Any history of fever?
- Are you taking any antibiotics?
- How long have the symptoms persisted?
- Any history of fever?
- Any history of headache and its location?
- Any history of dizziness or vertigo?

SORE THROAT

1. **How long have you had this?**

   [Time of onset is very important, especially when considering epiglottitis.]

2. **Have you had fever?**

   [The most common cause of sore throat is infection.]

3. **Have you had any drooling or difficulty swallowing saliva?**

   [These symptoms may indicate a more serious process, like peritonsillar abscess or epiglottitis. In small children, consider foreign body.]

4. **Are you a smoker?**

   [Persistent sore throat that does not respond to medication may indicate malignancy.]

5. **Have you had any difficulty breathing?**

   [This complaint is very serious! Consider peritonsillar abscess or epiglottitis.]

6. **Is anyone else at home sick?**

   [Consider infection spread by family members. The patient will often state that spouse, siblings, or other family members have similar symptoms.]

7. **Any significant past medical history?**

   [Of particular importance here is any history of thyroid disease or leukemia.]

8. **Have you noticed any sores or lesions on the tongue, lips, or gums?**

   [Painful mouth sores ("canker sores") may cause the patient to come to the Emergency Room complaining of "sore throat."]

9. **Are you taking any medications, antibiotics, or antivirals?**

   [Patients who are immunocompromised may be taking medications that cause oral candida.]

10. **Have you recently eaten anything new that you never had before?**

    [Consider allergic reaction.]

11. **Did you notice any tingling or a weird sensation around the mouth or lips before the sore throat?**

    [Herpes simplex type I may present with a prodrome of "tingling."]

12. **Any history of laryngitis or hoarseness or change in the voice?**

    [These symptoms may be caused by viral or bacterial infection, trauma with secondary edema of vocal cords, vocal nodes (singer's nodes), or malignancy.]

13. **Do you engage in oral sex?**

    [Consider papillomas, syphilis, or gonorrhea.]

14. **Have you felt unusually tired or "beat up"?**

    [Patients with Epstein Barr or "mono" will complain of sore throat and a feeling of increased generalized fatigue and body aches. These patients may present like a "flu" patient.]

15. **Have you noticed any rash with the sore throat?**

    [Patients with measles or scarlet fever may present with sore throat.]

DON'T FORGET TO ASK:

- Any history of fever?
- Symptoms of drooling
- Significant past medical history
- History of smoking
- Onset of symptoms
- Difficulty breathing

SYNCOPE

1. Do you have any significant family history, like heart disease or diabetes?

[A positive response suggests cardiac or other systemic illnesses, particularly a family history of arrhythmias or sudden death.]

2. Do you have any medical problems?

[Patients with coronary artery disease, left ventricular dysfunction, right ventricular dysplasia, diabetes, congestive heart failure, angina, and a positive cardiac history increase the likelihood of cardiac origin.]

3. Was there anyone with you when you fainted?

[Witnesses may report that the patient exhibited tongue biting, incontinence, or disorientation after syncope, which suggests seizure rather than syncope.]

4. Are you taking any medications?

[Alpha adrenergic blockers and nitrates, diuretics, tricyclic antidepressants, angiotensin-converting enzyme inhibitors, digoxin, to name a few. All may predispose to syncope.]

5. Have you had a recent change in your medication?

[A new medication or combination of medications may precipitate a syncopal episode.]

6. Does this happen a lot?

[Patients with multiple recurrent syncopal episodes over a period of months to years are at low risk for sudden cardiac death. These episodes are most likely vagal.]

7. **Did you have sweating or nausea either before or immediately after fainting?**

   [This is typical of a neurocardiogenic cause rather than ventricular arrhythmias or atrioventricular block.]

8. **Did you have blurred vision, double vision, or headache before the fainting episode?**

   [These symptoms strongly point to a neurologic cause.]

9. **Did this happen suddenly? Did you just black out without warning?**

   [Acute sudden syncope, without warning, suggests heart block or ventricular arrhythmia.]

10. **Did you have headache before fainting?**

    [Syncope preceded by headache may result from a migraine or intracerebral bleed. It may also be a vasovagal response.]

11. **Any shortness of breath or difficulty breathing?**

    [This suggests pulmonary embolism, pneumothorax, or hyperventilation.]

12. **Did you smell anything "funny" or see lights?**

    [A premonitory aura should lead to suspicion of a seizure.]

13. **Did you have a feeling of weakness or tingling in your arms or legs?**

    [Neurologic abnormalities are associated with seizures, migraines, strokes, or hyperventilation.]

14. **Were you shaving, tying a tie, or wearing a tight collar?**

    [Associated with carotid sinus syncope.]

15. **Did this happen immediately after eating?**

    [Syncope during or after meals is characteristic of postprandial or deglutition reflex syncope.]

16. **Did this happen while lying down?**

    [Cardiogenic syncope is suggested in any patient who experiences abrupt onset when supine.]

17. **Do you feel dizzy or like you are going to faint if you go from sitting to standing?**

    [This suggests orthostatic hypertension, which may be related to cardiac medications, exercise, or volume depletion.]

18. **Have you noticed dark stools or blood in your stool?**

    [Blood loss that can lead to anemia may cause secondary syncope.]

19. **Any history of fibroids or very heavy periods?**

    [Again, menorrhagia may lead to anemia and secondary syncope.]

20. **Were you exercising or doing anything strenuous when this happened?**

    [This would suggest cardiac outflow obstruction, which may be caused by aortic or sub-aortic stenosis, mitral stenosis, or cardiomyopathy.]

21. **Any history of chronic cough or bronchitis?**

    [Post-tussive syncope.]

22. **Any history of injury or trauma before the event?**

    [Especially head or chest blunt trauma.]

23. **Did you eat today?**

    [Simple hypoglycemia may lead to syncope.]

24. **Did you have chest pain?**

    [Myocardial infarction, pulmonary embolism, or metabolic syncope.]

25. **Have you been under more stress than usual from school work, boyfriend/girlfriend, spouse, or kids?**

    [Suggests vasovagal or neurocardiogenic origin.]

26. **Have you recently noticed tremor, weakness on one side, or changes in your vision?**

    [This suggests a neurologic problem.]

27. **Were you urinating when this happened?**

    [Patients with a history of obstructive urinary symptoms and syncope during or soon after vomiting may have micturition syncope.]

DON'T FORGET TO ASK:

- Loss of consciousness
- Past medical history
- Medications
- Chest pain
- Shortness of breath
- History of headache

URINARY TRACT INFECTION AND URINARY COMPLAINTS

Recurrent or frequent
UTI may warrant
broader antimicrobial
therapy.

1. **When did the symptoms first begin?**

   [Onset of symptoms may give clues to organisms involved.]

2. **Does it hurt or burn at the end of urinating?**

   [Simple noncomplicated urinary tract infection (UTI); consider sexually transmitted disease (STD), especially chlamydia.]

3. **Are you urinating more than usual?**

   [Frequency is a common complaint in UTI. Also ask the patient if they still feel as though they have to void again immediately after voiding.]

Pregnant women may
have asymptomatic UTI.

4. **Have you noticed any blood in the urine or change in color of urine?**

   [Hematuria coupled with back pain may indicate nephrolithiasis. Also, ask the female patient if she is menstruating.]

5. **Any abdominal pain? Show me with one finger where pain began.**

   [Patient with simple urinary tract infection may complain of suprapubic discomfort. Also consider possible sexually transmitted disease.]

Be careful: UTI in young
men may be
manifestation of
chlamydia infection.

6. **Have you had any back pain?**

   [Patients with nephrolithiasis or pyelonephritis may complain of back pain.]

7. **Any fever or chills?**

   [What initially looks like a simple uncomplicated UTI may be pyelonephritis in the making.]

8. **Do you have an active sex life?**

   [Consider "honeymoon cystitis."]

> Keep your index of suspicion up in children who present with UTI.

9. **Do you get this often?**

   [You may need to adjust treatment based on recurrence.]

10. **Have you had any abnormal vaginal discharge?**

    [Consider chlamydial urethritis.]

11. **Have you used any perfumed vaginal sprays or powders?**

    [These preparations can change pH of vaginal and urethral mucosa.]

12. **Have you over the last 5 days had oral sex?**

    [In women, oral sex may be contributing factor to UTI.]

13. **Have you had any dribbling at time of urination?**

    [In men consider benign, prostatic hypertrophy, prostatitis, urethral strictures.]

14. **Any pain in the groin?**

    [Consider STD, prostatitis, orchitis, or epididymitis.]

15. **Any change in the mental status?**

    [UTI in the elderly may initially manifest with confusion.]

16. **When you urinate do you wipe from front to back or back to front?**

    [It is especially important in women because wiping from back to front increases the possibility of introducing flora from the rectum to vagina.]

17. **Is it possible that you are drinking more water than usual?**

    [Always consider the obvious.]

DON'T FORGET TO ASK:

- Any history of fever
- In the elderly, always ask about change in mental status
- Is there back pain associated with symptoms?
- About dysuria, urgency, frequency
- About abdominal pain

VAGINAL BLEEDING

1. When was your last normal period?

[Normal is important because many patients, especially young patients, will consider any vaginal bleeding as "a normal period." This question also becomes important with peri-menopausal/premenopausal patients. Also consider pregnancy (ectopic or otherwise) or ovulation.]

Always be sure to check the cycle of the patient. In some instances the patient will lose track and present with a normal period.

2. How long have you had this bleeding?

[Sudden onset of vaginal bleeding may indicate pregnancy or trauma. However, prolonged vaginal bleeding may be caused by uterine myoma, dysfunctional uterine bleeding, or malignancy.]

3. Is this bleeding or spotting?

[The symptom of frank bright red bleeding may indicate incomplete abortion, inevitable abortion, menorrhagia, leiomyoma, normal menses, or dysfunctional uterine bleeding, whereas spotting may indicate ectopic pregnancy, cervical polyp, or dysfunctional uterine bleeding. Depending on age of the patient, both frank bleeding or spotting may indicate malignancy. Many hormonal imbalances will present this way; again, *always* consider the age of the patient.]

A complaint of spotting, pain, and a positive pregnancy test may indicate ectopic pregnancy.

4. Is bleeding painful or painless?

[Pain with bleeding may suggest endometriosis, leiomyoma, ectopic pregnancy, abortion, dysmenorrhea, or malignancy.]

Be sure to rule out foreign body or use of sexual objects during sex; forceful or vigorous sex play may cause injury and bleeding.

Know your population. Do not be afraid to use the word "pee." The vernacular may be the only thing standing between you and a good history.

Do not assume anything about your patient.

5. **Were you having sex when bleeding occurred?**

   [Postcoital or coital bleeding may indicate cervical polyp, malignancy, cervical dysplasia, or in the older patient may be a result of atrophic vaginitis.]

6. **Have you recently had any procedures?**

   [Consider recent termination of pregnancy, dilation and curettage, retained products of contraception, cryo, loop electrosurgical excision procedure, vaginal hysterectomy/abdominal hysterectomy, cervical or vaginal radiation. In rare instances, consider arterial venous malformation.]

7. **Is bleeding constant or off and on?**

   [Although rare, bleeding that alternates between being very heavy one moment and then very light may indicate arterial venous malformation, especially if symptoms occur after a procedure.]

8. **Does it hurt or burn when you urinate? Are you going more than usual?**

   [Urinary tract infection may give a symptom of spotting.]

9. **Do you notice the blood in your panties or when you wipe yourself?**

   [If bleeding is only noticeable when wiping after urinating, urinary tract infection or hemorrhoids are indicated.]

10. **Is there any odor associated with the bleeding?**

    [Foul-smelling vaginal bleeding may be associated with infection, foreign body, or malignancy.]

11. **Have you noticed any clotting?**

    [Consider incomplete abortion, leiomyoma or blood dyscrasias.]

12. **Is there any chance that you are pregnant?**

    [Bleeding in early pregnancy may indicate a threatening abortion or, if associated with pain, ectopic pregnancy.]

13. **Do you have any other medical problems?**

[Older women who present with vaginal bleeding and are diabetic, hypertensive, and/or obese may be set up for endometrial cancer. ALWAYS CONSIDER SYSTEMIC DISEASE.]

14. **Are you taking any medications, including vitamins and oral contraceptives?**

[Aside from anticoagulants, vitamin E may "thin" the blood. Oral contraceptives may also contribute to menorrhagia/metrorrhagia.]

15. **Are you sure bleeding is from vagina?**

[Many times the patient will complain of vaginal bleeding when in fact the bleeding is coming from hemorrhoids or the urethra.]

16. **When was your last Pap smear?**

[Again, cervical dysplasia or malignancy may contribute to vaginal bleeding.]

17. **How old were you when you got your first period?**

[This is important when you want to rule out dysfunctional or anovulatory bleeding.]

18. **Are you having protected sex? Are you using condoms?**

[Patients having unprotected sex increase their risks of exposure to sexually transmitted diseases, such as human papilloma virus and trichomoniasis; both may lead to cervical dysplasia and vaginal bleeding, particularly postcoital.]

19. **Are your periods usually regular and on time?**

[Always rule out possibility that this may be a "normal" menses.]

20. **Any history of gonorrhea or chlamydia?**

[Female patients who have a history of gonorrhea or chlamydia may have tubo-ovarian adhesions, increasing the risk of ectopic pregnancy.]

21. Have you ever been admitted to the hospital for any infection in your tubes?

[These patients are more likely to develop ectopic pregnancy.]

22. Any history of surgery on your belly?

[Again, patients who have undergone abdominal surgery are predisposed to ectopic pregnancy.]

DON'T FORGET TO ASK:

- When was the last normal period?
- How long has bleeding been going on?
- Are the sanitary pads saturated and how often they need to be changed?
- Last sexually active
- Has this ever happened before?

VAGINAL DISCHARGE

1. How long have you had discharge?

[The incubation period varies with pathology. Generally, the incubation period for most sexually transmitted diseases (STDs) is 7 to 14 days. However, with genital warts this period may extend to 7 to 18 days.]

Homosexual patients who have never had a heterosexual relationship do not present with pathology typically found in heterosexuals.

2. Is this discharge abnormal to you?

[Any woman of childbearing age will have a "normal" odorless clear to whitish discharge.]

3. When was your last normal period?

[Consistency and color of vaginal discharge will change with the phases of the menstrual cycle; during the luteal phase, the discharge may become copious, thick, and mucoid. During the ovulatory phase, consistency may change to white, odorless, and pasty.]

We live in a wonderfully diverse world. Do not assume your patient is heterosexual.

4. When was the last time that you had sex?

[Again, the time of last intercourse may directly correlate with onset of symptoms.]

5. Are you heterosexual?

[Homosexual women, who have never had a heterosexual experience, very rarely develop STDs.]

6. Does the discharge have an odor?

[If the discharge is odorless, you have already ruled out bacterial vaginosis, which is characteristically "fishy." If particularly foul, suspect foreign body.]

Do not be afraid to ask your patient pointed questions.

7. What color is the discharge?

[Remember, it is normal for young women to have a clear to whitish discharge. Suspect a problem if discharge is yellow to tan or brownish.]

8. Does the discharge cause itching?

[Typically, trichomoniasis does not itch. There can be considerable itching with candidiasis or genital herpes.]

9. Has your partner had any symptoms?

[This will assist in narrowing your diagnosis. However, because chlamydia may be asymptomatic, maintain your suspicions. Both patient and partner should be treated.]

10. Have you ever had this discharge before?

[Patients with multiple hospital evaluations for STD may need to be treated more aggressively.]

11. Did you use condoms the last time that you had sex?

[If the patient is using condoms, this will narrow your diagnosis for possible causes of the vaginal discharge.]

12. Is this a new partner?

[If patient has been asymptomatic until having intercourse with a new partner, this increases the likelihood of an STD.]

13. Do you use tampons?

[Be very careful when prescribing medications. Surprisingly so, a large number of women, particularly young women, are afraid to touch or put anything in the vagina.]

DON'T FORGET TO ASK:

- Did the patient have sex before the onset of symptoms?
- About history of medication, birth control pills, over the counter products
- Significant past medical history
- Is there itching with the discharge?

VAGINAL ITCHING

Consider your patient's age; atrophic vaginitis may also cause itching.

1. **How long have you had the itching?**

[Vaginal itching that is acute may be related to candida, genital herpes, or contact dermatitis. Prolonged intractable vaginal itching in the older woman that does not respond to medication may indicate malignancy.]

2. **Do you have any vaginal burning?**

[May indicate genital herpes, candida, or urinary tract pathology.]

3. **Do you have any discharge with the itching?**

Always begin your history with "how long have symptoms been present?"

[Candida is typically thick and white. However, candida may be present with an atypical presentation. Typically, trichomoniasis or bacterial vaginosis may not cause pruritus.]

4. **What color?**

[The discharge associated with candida is typically thick, while trichomoniasis is thin, copious and greenish/yellow. Normal vaginal discharge is clear to pasty white and is not malodorous.]

5. **Does discharge have odor?**

[Foul-smelling vaginal discharge may indicate bacterial vaginosis.]

Itching and irritation are perceived as the same symptom in patients.

6. **When is the last time that you had sex?**

[Incubation period important here.]

7. **Do you use condoms? Or spermicidal foams or jelly?**

[A large number of women are allergic to nonoxynol 9, which is present in spermicides. This may lead to vaginal irritation.]

8. Have you been douching?

[Douching alters the pH of the vagina and can cause vaginal irritation as do other so-called feminine hygiene products like perfumed suppositories, sprays, lotions, and powders.]

> Keep in mind incubation period for various disease processes.

9. Have you recently had oral sex?

[Oral sex can alter the pH of the vagina, leading to development of candidiasis.]

10. Have you used over the counter preparations for cure?

[Many over the counter preparations will actually increase the patient's symptoms of itching and irritation.]

> Know your population. Do not be afraid to use words that the patient understands.

11. Have you used any powders, perfumes, lotions, or feminine hygiene deodorants?

[These products may cause vaginal irritation and itching.]

12. Have you changed sanitary pads or recently switched to tampons?

[Many sanitary pads and tampons are made with synthetic fibers and may irritate sensitive vaginal tissue.]

> In some instances, even the vernacular is accepted. Do not assume that your patient knows what "oral sex" is.

13. Do you have any medical problems?

[Women with diabetes may have frequent candida infections. In fact, vaginal candidiasis may be the first sign of new onset diabetes.]

14. Do you use tampons or pads?

[Some women may be allergic to the synthetic fibers of some pads or the string attached to the tampon.]

15. Are you taking antibiotics or oral contraceptives?

[Both may alter pH of the vagina and cause overgrowth of yeast, leading to itching and irritation.]

16. Any abnormal discharge?

[Abnormal is key, because many women of childbearing age will have a normal discharge.]

17. Do you have pain in the vagina?

[Pain in the vagina may indicate genital herpes, excoriation secondary to candida, or psychological disturbance.]

18. Any groin pain?

[May indicate inguinal adenopathy.]

19. Any sores or lesions on the vagina associated with the itching?

[Sores or lesions on the vagina that are painful are usually associated with genital herpes, whereas painless lesions may indicate first-degree syphilis or chancroid.]

DON'T FORGET TO ASK:

- Did the patient have sex before onset of symptoms?
- About history of medications, birth control pills, over the counter products
- Significant past medical history
- Is there pain with the itching?

WRIST INJURIES

1. **Any history of injury or trauma?**

   [Most wrist injuries result from a fall on the outstretched hand.]

2. **Has this ever happened before?**

   [Previous wrist injuries are important because of possible ongoing ligamentous instability, like distal radioulnar joint laxity.]

3. **What kind of work do you do? Are you into sports?**

   [In overuse injuries, often there is no history of trauma but a pattern of repetitive use in daily work or home activity.]

4. **Is this your dominant hand?**

   [Disability is greater when the dominant wrist is injured.]

5. **Do you have any significant past medical history?**

   [Particularly collagen vascular disease, diabetes, or immunosuppression, all of which impede healing.]

6. **Does it hurt you to flex the wrist?**

   [If the patient complains of increased pain with flexion of the wrist, this may indicate a fracture or carpal dislocation.]

7. **Any pain in the side of the wrist?**

   [Pain in the *"snuff box"* area, coupled with pain that is increased with axial loading of the thumb, should alert you to a possible navicular fracture.]

8. **What were you doing when this happened?**

   [Be alert for hamate fractures, which occur especially in athletes. This type of fracture is suggested when a bat or club is held and struck against an immovable object.]

DON'T FORGET TO ASK:

- What were you doing when this happened?
- Any significant past medical history
- If the pain is increased with specific movement
- Has this ever happened before?

INDEX

Abdominal distention, 4, 73
Abdominal pain, 1–6
  and back pain, 3, 12, 14
  and chest pain, 3, 22, 25
  and eye complaints, 52
  and fainting, 3, 83
  and fever, 1, 2, 54
  and loss of consciousness, 83
  in motor vehicle accidents, 71
  in nausea and vomiting, 1, 72
  sexual history in, 5, 87, 91
  and shoulder pain, 3, 94
  and stool changes, 4, 28
  in urinary tract disorders, 4, 104, 106
    in hematuria, 4, 63, 64
    in nephrolithiasis, 2, 3, 4
Abrasions, 68–69
Acromioclavicular joint dislocation, 93
Alcohol use, gastrointestinal bleeding in, 29
Allergy history
  in ankle injuries, 10
  in bite wounds, 15
  in breathing difficulty, 38
  in burns, 17, 18
  in lacerations and abrasions, 68, 69
  in needlestick injuries, 75
  in rash, 79, 80
  in seizures and loss of consciousness, 84
  in sexual assault, 88
Anemia
  in diarrhea, 30
  oral complaints in, 77
  syncope in, 83, 84, 102
Aneurysm of aorta, 29
  abdominal pain in, 2, 3
  back pain in, 11, 12
Angina
  Ludwig's, 78
  pectoris, 21, 23, 24
  Prinzmetal's variant, 24

  Vincent's, 76
Ankle injuries, 9–10
Anorexia, 35
Antibiotics
  in ankle injuries, 10
  in bite wounds, 15
  in burns, 17
  in sinusitis, 97
Anxiety, 35–36
Aorta
  aneurysm of, 29
    abdominal pain in, 2, 3
    back pain in, 11, 12
  dissection of, chest pain in, 22, 23
Appendicitis
  abdominal pain in, 1, 2, 3, 4, 6
  nausea and vomiting in, 72
Appetite changes, 27
  in fever, 55
  and loss of consciousness, 84
  in psychological disorders, 35
Arteriosclerosis obliterans, calf pain in, 19
Arteritis, temporal, 51, 52, 58, 61
Arthritis, 65–67
  and eye complaints, 52
  and fever, 55, 56
  and inflammatory bowel disease, 30
Ascites, 46
Assault, sexual, 86–89
Asthma, 32, 33, 34
Aura
  in migraine, 60
  in seizures, 83, 85, 101

Back pain, 11–14
  and abdominal pain, 3, 12, 14
  and chest pain, 13, 22, 25
  and fever, 13, 14, 54
  and hematuria, 12, 104
  and loss of consciousness, 83

Back pain, *continued*
  in motor vehicle accidents, 71
  in urinary tract disorders, 11, 12, 13, 104,
    106
Barotrauma
  dizziness in, 42
  ear complaints in, 44
Bismuth poisoning, 76
Bites, 15–16
  fever in, 16, 55
  rash in, 79, 80
Bladder infections, 63, 105
Bowel function, 26–30
  in abdominal pain, 4
  in back pain, 13
  in motor vehicle accidents, 71
Brain tumors, headache in, 59, 60, 61
Breathing difficulty, 37–39
  and abdominal pain, 3
  and back pain, 12
  in burns, 17
  and calf pain, 20
  and chest pain, 21, 24, 37, 38
  in edema, 38, 46, 47
  in fever, 37, 55
  in motor vehicle accidents, 71
  and shoulder pain, 94, 95
  in sore throat, 98, 99
  syncope in, 101
Burns, 17–18
Bursitis, shoulder pain in, 95

Calculi, renal, 104
  abdominal pain in, 2, 3, 4
  back pain in, 11
Calf pain, 19–20
Cardiovascular disorders
  breathing difficulty in, 37, 38, 39
  chest pain in, 21–25
    and syncope, 24, 83, 102, 103
  cough in, 31, 32, 33
  dizziness in, 40, 41
  edema in, 46, 47
  seizures and loss of consciousness in, 83
  syncope in, 100, 101, 102
    and chest pain, 24, 83, 102, 103
    onset of, 41, 101
Carotid sinus syncope, 101
Cauda equina syndrome, back pain in, 13
Cellulitis
  calf pain in, 19, 20
  orbital, 52, 53
Cerebrovascular disorders
  dizziness in, 41
  headache in, 8, 58, 60, 62, 101

  seizures and loss of consciousness in, 82,
    83
Chemical exposure
  breathing difficulty in, 39
  burns in, 17
  cough in, 32
Chest pain, 21–25
  and abdominal pain, 3, 22, 25
  and back pain, 13, 22, 25
  and breathing difficulty, 21, 24, 37, 38
  and cough, 31, 34
  and fever, 21, 55
  and loss of consciousness, 83
  psychological factors in, 21, 36
  and syncope, 24, 83, 102, 103
Children
  breathing difficulty in, 38
  cough in, 33
  ear complaints in, 45
  epistaxis in, 49
  rash in, 80, 81
  sexual assault of, 88–89
  shoulder pain in, 93
  sore throat in, 98
  urinary tract infections in, 105
Chlamydial infections, 90, 92
  abdominal pain in, 5
  urinary complaints in, 104, 105
  vaginal bleeding in, 109
  vaginal discharge in, 112
Cholecystitis, 2, 11, 12
Cholesteatoma, 43, 44
Colitis, 26, 27, 28
Colorectal cancer, 27, 28
Conjunctivitis, 50, 51
Consciousness, loss of, 82–85
  in motor vehicle accidents, 70, 71
  in sexual assault, 88, 89
  in syncope, 100–103
Constipation, 26–30
Costochondritis, chest pain in, 22
Cough, 31–34
  and breathing difficulty, 38
  and eye complaints, 53
  and fever, 31, 54
  and gastrointestinal bleeding, 29
  and syncope, 102
Crohn's disease, 27, 28
Cyst, ovarian, 5, 6
Cystitis, 63, 105

Depression, 35–36
Dermatitis, contact, 79, 80
Diabetic retinopathy, 50, 51
Diarrhea, 26–30

Discharge
  from ear, 44
  from penis, 90, 92
  from vagina, 111–113. *See also* Vagina,
    discharge from
Diverticulitis, 27
Dizziness, 40–42, 100–103
  and abdominal pain, 3
  and chest pain, 24
  and diarrhea, 30
  and ear complaints, 41, 44, 45
  and headache, 40, 58
  in nausea and vomiting, 74
Dog bites, 15
Drug use history
  in abdominal pain, 2, 3, 5, 6
  in ankle injuries, 10
  in back pain, 11
  in bite wounds, 16
  in breathing difficulty, 37, 39
  in calf pain, 20
  in chest pain, 23, 24
  in cough, 31, 32, 34
  in dizziness, 41, 42
  in ear complaints, 43
  in edema, 46, 47
  in epistaxis, 48, 49
  in eye complaints, 52
  in fever, 55, 56, 57
  in gastrointestinal bleeding, 27, 29
  in headache, 59, 62
  in hematuria, 64
  in joint pain, 65
  in lacerations and abrasions, 69
  in mental status alteration, 7, 8
  in nausea and vomiting, 73
  in psychological disorders, 35, 36
  in rash, 79
  in seizures and loss of consciousness, 83,
    85
  in sexual assault, 88
  in sinusitis, 97
  in sore throat, 99
  in stool changes, 27, 29, 30
  in syncope, 100, 103
  in vaginal bleeding, 109
  in vaginal itching, 115, 116
Duodenal ulcer. *See* Ulcer of stomach and
    duodenum
Dyspnea, 37–38. *See also* Breathing
    difficulty

Ear complaints, 41, 43–45
  and dizziness, 41, 44, 45
  and fever, 43, 45, 54, 56

  in nausea and vomiting, 74
Eclampsia, 82
Ectopic pregnancy
  abdominal pain in, 1, 2, 3, 4, 5
  shoulder pain in, 94
  vaginal bleeding in, 107, 108, 109, 110
Edema, 46–47
  breathing difficulty in, 38, 46, 47
Elderly
  epistaxis in, 48
  lacerations and abrasions in, 68
  mental status alteration in, 7, 55, 105, 106
  psychological disorders in, 35
  seizures in, 82
  urinary tract infections in, 55, 105, 106
Endophthalmitis, 51, 52
Epididymitis, 91, 92, 105
Epiglottitis, 98
Epistaxis, 48–49
Eye complaints, 50–53
  and dizziness, 41
  and fainting, 101
  and headache, 52, 58, 60, 61, 62
  in nausea and vomiting, 74

Fainting, 82–85, 100–103
  and abdominal pain, 3, 83
  and diarrhea, 30
  and headache, 60, 101
  in nausea and vomiting, 74, 101
Family history
  in abdominal pain, 5, 6
  in chest pain, 23
  in cough, 33
  in diarrhea, 28
  in epistaxis, 48
  in headache, 58, 59
  in joint pain, 65
  in sore throat, 98
  in suicide attempt, 36
  in syncope, 100
Fever, 54–57
  and abdominal pain, 1, 2, 54
  and back pain, 13, 14, 54
  and bite wounds, 16, 55
  and breathing difficulty, 37, 55
  and calf pain, 19, 20
  and chest pain, 21, 55
  and cough, 31, 54
  and ear complaints, 43, 45, 54, 56
  and edema, 46
  and eye complaints, 52
  and headache, 58
  and joint pain, 55, 56, 65, 67
  and mental status alteration, 8, 55

Fever, *continued*
  nausea and vomiting in, 72, 74
  and oral complaints, 76
  and rash, 79, 81
  and seizures, 82
  and sexually transmitted diseases, 55, 92
  and sinusitis, 96, 97
  and sore throat, 98, 99
  and urinary tract disorders, 54, 104, 106
Fibroids, uterine, 5, 13
Flatulence
  and abdominal pain, 4
  and breathing difficulty, 39
  and chest pain, 22
Food poisoning
  abdominal pain in, 1, 5
  diarrhea in, 28
  nausea and vomiting in, 72, 73
Foreign bodies
  breathing difficulty in, 38
  cough in, 33
  in ear, 43
  epistaxis in, 49
  in lacerations and abrasions, 68, 69
  vaginal bleeding in, 107, 108
Fractures
  in ankle injuries, 9, 10
  back pain in, 11, 13
  shoulder pain in, 93, 94
  in wrist injuries, 117–118

Gastroesophageal reflux
  back pain in, 13
  breathing difficulty in, 38, 39
  cough in, 31, 32, 33, 34
Gastrointestinal disorders, 26–30
  abdominal pain in, 1, 2, 3
  back pain in, 13
  breathing difficulty in, 38, 39
  chest pain in, 22, 23, 25
  cough in, 31, 32, 33, 34
  nausea and vomiting, 72–74. *See also*
    Nausea and vomiting
  ulcer of stomach and duodenum. *See*
    Ulcer of stomach and duodenum
Gingival disorders, 76–78
  and sinusitis, 96
Glaucoma, 50, 51, 52
  nausea and vomiting in, 74
Glenohumeral joint disorders, 93–95
Glomerulonephritis, hematuria in, 63, 64
Gonorrhea, 90
  abdominal pain in, 5
  anorectal, 27, 29, 91
  joint pain in, 67, 92

sore throat in, 98, 99
  vaginal bleeding in, 109
Gout, 65, 66, 67
Groin pain
  and abdominal pain, 3
  in sexually transmitted diseases, 91
  and urinary complaints, 105
  and vaginal itching, 116

Hand injuries, 117–118
  in bites, 15–16
Head injury
  eye complaints in, 50, 52
  in motor vehicle accidents, 70, 71
  seizures in, 83
  in sexual assault, 86, 88
Headache, 58–62
  in burns, 17
  in cerebrovascular disorders, 8, 58, 60,
    62, 101
  and dizziness, 40, 58
  and eye complaints, 52, 58, 60, 61, 62
  and fainting, 60, 101
  in sinusitis, 60, 96, 97
  and syncope, 60, 101, 103
Hearing loss, 43–45
  and dizziness, 41, 42
Heart failure
  breathing difficulty in, 37, 38, 39
  cough in, 31, 32, 33
  edema in, 46, 47
Hematemesis, 27
Hematochezia, 26
Hematoma, subdural, headache in, 60, 62
Hematuria, 63–64, 104
  and abdominal pain, 4, 63, 64
  and back pain, 12, 104
Hemoptysis, 32
Hemorrhage
  epistaxis in, 48–49
  gastrointestinal, 26, 27, 28, 29
  hematuria in, 4, 12, 63–64, 104
  in lacerations and abrasions, 69
  vaginal, 5, 63, 107–110
Hemorrhoids, 26, 29, 108, 109
Hepatitis
  in needlestick injuries, 75
  in sexual assault, 88
Herbal preparations
  in chest pain, 23
  in joint pain, 65
HIV infection and AIDS
  cough in, 32, 33
  lacerations and abrasions in, 69
  in needlestick injuries, 75

Hyperthermia, malignant, 54
Hypotension, postural, 41, 67, 102

Infarction, myocardial
  back pain in, 13
  chest pain in, 21, 23, 24, 25
Infections
  abdominal pain in, 1, 2, 3, 5
  in ankle injuries, 10
  back pain in, 12, 13
  in bite wounds, 15, 16
  breathing difficulty in, 37
  cough in, 31, 32, 33
  diarrhea in, 26, 27, 28
  dizziness in, 40
  ear complaints in, 43, 45
  eye complaints in, 50, 51, 52, 53
  fever in, 54–57
  headache in, 58
  hematuria in, 63, 64
  joint pain in, 65, 67
  in lacerations and abrasions, 68, 69
  mental status alteration in, 8
  nausea and vomiting in, 72
  oral complaints in, 76, 77
  rash in, 79, 80
  sexually transmitted, 90–92
  sinusitis in, 96–97
  sore throat in, 98–99
  of urinary tract, 104–106
  vaginal discharge in, 111–113
  vaginal itching in, 114
Inflammatory bowel disease, 26, 27, 28, 30
Inhalation injuries, 17
Irritable bowel syndrome, 26, 27
Itching
  of ear, 45
  of eyes, 51
  in rash, 79
  in sexually transmitted diseases, 91
  vaginal, 114–116
    with vaginal discharge, 112, 113, 114, 115

Joint pain, 65–67
  and fever, 55, 56, 65, 67
  and rash, 79, 81
  in sexually transmitted diseases, 67, 92

Kidney disorders, 104
  abdominal pain in, 2, 3, 4
  back pain in, 11, 12
  hematuria in, 63, 64

Labyrinthitis, 40, 41, 44

Lacerations, 68–69
Laryngitis, 76, 99
Lead poisoning, 76
Leg, calf pain in, 19–20
Leiomyoma of uterus
  abdominal pain in, 5
  back pain in, 13
  vaginal bleeding in, 107, 108
Leukemia, oral complaints in, 77
Light sensitivity in eye complaints, 50, 52
Liver disorders
  bite wounds in, 15
  edema in, 46
  hepatitis, 75, 88
Ludwig's angina, 78
Lymphedema, calf pain in, 20

Mallory-Weiss syndrome, 27, 29
Marijuana use, cough in, 31, 32
Medication history. *See* Drug use history
Meigs' syndrome, 4, 73
Melena, 26–30
Ménière's disease
  dizziness in, 40, 41, 42
  ear complaints in, 41, 43, 44, 45
Menorrhagia, 83, 102, 107
Menstrual history, 107–109
  in abdominal pain, 4, 5
  in chest pain, 24
  in hematuria, 64, 104
  in shoulder pain, 94
  in syncope, 83, 102
Mental status alteration, 7–8
  and fever, 8, 55
  and urinary tract infection, 55, 105, 106
Migraine, 58, 60, 61
Mononucleosis, 77, 99
Motor vehicle accidents, 70–71
Mouth disorders, 76–78
  and sinusitis, 96, 97
  and sore throat, 98
Multiple sclerosis, dizziness in, 40, 41
Munchausen's syndrome, 63
Myocardial infarction
  back pain in, 13
  chest pain in, 21, 23, 24, 25

Nausea and vomiting, 72–74
  abdominal pain in, 1, 72
  back pain in, 12
  in burns, 17
  chest pain in, 21, 25
  dizziness in, 40
  ear complaints in, 44
  eye complaints in, 52

Nausea and vomiting, *continued*
  fainting in, 74, 101
  headache in, 58, 60, 62
  hematemesis in, 27
Needlestick injuries, 75
Nephrolithiasis, 104
  abdominal pain in, 2, 3, 4
  back pain in, 11
Neuroma, acoustic, 41, 42
Nosebleeds, 48–49

Odor
  of breath, 76
  of ear, 43, 44
  of stool, 26
  of vaginal discharge, 90, 108, 111, 114
Oral complaints, 76–78
  and sinusitis, 96, 97
  and sore throat, 98
Orchitis, 91, 92, 105
Otitis, 43, 44, 45
Ovarian disorders, abdominal pain in, 1, 4,
    5, 6
Over the counter preparations
  in abdominal pain, 2, 3
  in chest pain, 23, 24
  in headache, 59
  in joint pain, 65
  in vaginal itching, 115

Pain
  abdominal, 1–6. *See also* Abdominal pain
  in back, 11–14. *See also* Back pain
  in bites, 16
  in calf, 19–20
  in chest, 21–25. *See also* Chest pain
  in ear, 43–45
  in edema, 47
  in eye, 50, 51, 52, 53
  in groin. *See* Groin pain
  in headache, 58–62. *See also* Headache
  in joints, 65–67. *See also* Joint pain
  in shoulder, 93–95
    and abdominal pain, 3, 94
  in urination. *See* Urination, pain in
  in vaginal bleeding, 107
  in vaginal itching, 116
  in wrist, 117–118
Pancreatitis, abdominal pain in, 2, 3, 6
Panic disorder, 36
Papilloma, sore throat in, 98, 99
Pelvic inflammatory disease, abdominal
    pain in, 3
Penile discharge in sexually transmitted
    diseases, 90, 92

Pericarditis, chest pain in, 21, 22, 25
Pharyngitis, 76, 98
Photophobia, 50, 52
Plummer-Vinson syndrome, 77
Pneumonia
  chest pain in, 21
  cough in, 31, 32, 33
Posture
  in abdominal pain, 2
  in breathing difficulty, 37, 38
  in calf pain, 19
  in chest pain, 22
  in dizziness, 41
  in headache, 60
  in seizures and loss of consciousness, 84
  in sinusitis, 96
  in syncope, 84, 101, 102
Pregnancy
  abdominal pain in, 1, 2, 3, 4, 5
  ectopic. *See* Ectopic pregnancy
  hematuria in, 63
  nausea and vomiting in, 72, 73, 74
  seizures in, 82, 83, 85
  shoulder pain in, 94
  urinary tract infections in, 104
  vaginal bleeding in, 107, 108, 109, 110
Proctitis, 28, 29
Prostate disorders, 105
Psychological factors, 35–36
  in abdominal pain, 4
  in breathing difficulty, 39
  in chest pain, 21, 36
  in dizziness, 40
  in edema, 47
  in headache, 58, 59
Pyelonephritis, 12, 104

Rabies, 15, 16
Radiculopathy, back pain in, 13
Ramsay-Hunt syndrome, 44
Rash, 79–81
  in sexually transmitted diseases, 91
  and sore throat, 99
Rectal pain, 29, 91
Reflux, gastroesophageal. *See*
    Gastroesophageal reflux
Respiratory disorders
  breathing difficulty in, 37–39. *See also*
      Breathing difficulty
  cough in, 31–34. *See also* Cough
Retinal disorders, 50, 51, 52
Rheumatoid arthritis, 65, 66
Rotator cuff disorders, 93, 94, 95

Salpingitis, 5, 91, 92

Sciatica, 11
Sclerosis, multiple, 40, 41
Seizures, 82–85, 100, 101
  aura in, 83, 85, 101
  mental status alteration in, 7
Sexual assault, 86–89
Sexual history, 90–92
  in abdominal pain, 5, 87, 91
  in fever, 55, 92
  in joint pain, 67, 92
  in rectal pain, 29, 91
  sexual assault in, 86–89
  in sore throat, 98, 99
  in stool changes, 28, 29
  in urinary complaints, 90, 104, 105
  in vaginal bleeding, 107, 108, 109
  in vaginal discharge, 90, 92, 111, 112, 113
  in vaginal itching, 114, 115, 116
Shoulder pain, 93–95
  and abdominal pain, 3, 94
Sialolithiasis, 78
Sinusitis, 96–97
  eye complaints in, 52
  headache in, 60, 96, 97
Sleep problems
  in abdominal pain, 2
  in chest pain, 24
  in headache, 60, 61, 62
  in psychological disorders, 35
Smoking
  breathing difficulty in, 37, 39
  chest pain in, 22
  cough in, 32, 34
  dizziness in, 42
  edema in, 47
  headache in, 59
  oral complaints in, 76
  sore throat in, 98, 99
Spinal stenosis, 13
Spousal abuse, 6
Stomach ulcer. *See* Ulcer of stomach and
    duodenum
Stool changes, 26–30
  and abdominal pain, 4, 28
  in color, 26, 84, 102
  in odor, 26
Suicide attempt, 35–36
Surgical history
  in abdominal pain, 4
  in breathing difficulty, 39
  in edema, 47
  in eye complaints, 51, 52
  in fever, 54, 55
  in gastrointestinal bleeding, 29
  in hematuria, 64

  in nausea and vomiting, 73
  in vaginal bleeding, 108, 110
Sweating at night
  in cough, 32
  in fever, 56
Syncope, 83, 84, 100–103
  in anemia, 83, 84, 102
  in cardiovascular disorders, 83, 100, 101,
    102
    and chest pain, 24, 83, 102, 103
    onset of, 41, 101
  in diarrhea, 30
  and headache, 60, 101, 103
  menstrual history in, 83, 102
  position at time of, 84, 101, 102
Syphilis, 88, 91

Tampon use
  and vaginal discharge, 112
  and vaginal itching, 115
Temporal arteritis, 51, 52, 58, 61
Tenesmus, 27, 28
Testicular pain, 91
Tetanus prophylaxis
  in ankle injuries, 10
  in bites, 15, 16
  in burns, 17, 18
  in lacerations and abrasions, 68
  in needlestick injuries, 75
Throat, sore, 98–99
  and rash, 80, 81
Thrombophlebitis, calf pain in, 19, 20
Thrombosis, deep vein, calf pain in, 19, 20
Tinnitus, 45
Tongue disorders, 76–78
Tonsillitis, 76
Tooth disorders, 76–78
  and sinusitis, 96, 97
Trauma
  abdominal pain in, 3, 6
  ankle injuries in, 9–10
  back pain in, 11, 12, 14
  in bites, 15–16
  breathing difficulty in, 38
  in burns, 17–18
  chest pain in, 22, 24
  dizziness in, 41, 42
  ear complaints in, 43, 45
  edema in, 46
  epistaxis in, 48, 49
  eye complaints in, 50, 52
  headache in, 60
  hematuria in, 63, 64
  joint pain in, 66
  lacerations and abrasions in, 68–69

Trauma, *continued*
  mental status alteration in, 7
  in motor vehicle accidents, 70–71
  in needlestick injuries, 75
  seizures in, 83
  in sexual assault, 86–89
  shoulder pain in, 93, 94, 95
  sinusitis in, 97
  syncope in, 102
  of wrist, 117–118
Travel history
  in diarrhea, 28
  in dizziness, 42
  in ear complaints, 44
  in epistaxis, 48

Ulcer of stomach and duodenum
  abdominal pain in, 1, 2, 3
  chest pain in, 22, 23, 25
  nausea and vomiting in, 72, 73
Urinary tract disorders, 104–106
  abdominal pain in, 4, 104, 106
    in hematuria, 4, 63, 64
    in nephrolithiasis, 2, 3, 4
  back pain in, 11, 12, 13, 104, 106
  differentiated from vaginal disorders, 108,
    109
  in elderly, 55, 105, 106
  and eye complaints, 52
  fever in, 54, 104, 106
  hematuria in, 63–64, 104
    and abdominal pain, 4, 63, 64
    and back pain, 12, 104
  of kidneys. *See* Kidney disorders
  mental status alteration in, 55, 105, 106
  in motor vehicle accidents, 71
  sexual history in, 90, 104, 105
  syncope in, 103
Urination
  frequency of, 104, 108
    in eye complaints, 52
    in fever, 54
    in hematuria, 63
    in sexually transmitted diseases, 90
    in vaginal bleeding, 108
  pain in, 104
    in eye complaints, 52
    in fever, 54
    in hematuria, 63

    in sexually transmitted diseases, 90,
      104
    in vaginal bleeding, 108
  syncope in, 103
Urine
  blood in, 4, 12, 63–64, 104
  color of, 63, 104
Uterus
  bleeding from, dysfunctional, 107
  fibroids and leiomyoma of, 5, 13
    abdominal pain in, 5
    back pain in, 13
    vaginal bleeding in, 107, 108

Vagina
  bleeding from, 107–110
    abdominal pain in, 5
    hematuria in, 63
  discharge from, 105, 111–113
    abdominal pain in, 5
    color of, 90, 112, 114
    fever in, 56
    itching in, 112, 113, 114, 115
    odor of, 90, 108, 111, 114
    sexual history in, 90, 92, 111, 112,
      113
  itching of, 114–116
    discharge in, 112, 113, 114, 115
Varicose veins, calf pain in, 19, 20
Vertigo, 40–42
Vincent's angina, 76
Vision disorders, 50–53
  and dizziness, 41
  and fainting, 101
  and headache, 58, 60, 62
Vitamin B12 deficiency, oral complaints in,
  77
Vomiting. *See* Nausea and vomiting

Weight loss
  and abdominal pain, 4
  and cough, 32
  and fever, 56
  and stool changes, 28
Wrestling injuries
  abdominal pain in, 3, 6
  back pain in, 12
  chest pain in, 22
Wrist injuries, 117–118